"Peace Building through Health (PtH), the author, sounded like Peace Building through Hell. I did not attempt to question this, because what I heard applies to our reality under Israeli military occupation. After reading this amazing chronicle of an American organization trying to mitigate a hyper-sensitive political web for the sake of the health of both Palestinians and Israelis, I am confident that we all can be part of the solution if we so desire. One sentence in the book stood out, 'PtH is a political process.' HATD working at the community level is a clear confirmation of their politics of empowerment. This book goes behind the headlines and gives a hands-on taste of what so many must grapple with daily."

Sam Bahour, *Palestinian-American businessman, writer, activist, Al-Bireh/Ramallah, Palestine*

"As a health professional living and working in Israel all my adult life, I've been engaged in peace through health. Through the remarkable accomplishments of Healing Across the Divides, this book by Dr Goldfield highlights what are the possible roles of health professionals in the Israeli-Palestinian conflict. I highly recommend this book to all health professionals interested in this field and to all interested in knowing what is achievable in this challenging conflict."

Professor Raphael Walden, *President, Physicians for Human Rights–Israel; professor of medicine at Tel Aviv University*

"Healing Across the Divides, a U.S. nonprofit, provides small grants and back-up to small Palestinian and Jewish groups that face common health needs that lack government support. These low-overhead largely community groups run a variety of programs, e.g., diabetes, nutrition and obesity, that help tens of thousands, and create uncommon rapport and collaboration. As Israel and Palestine wrestle endlessly, and sometimes violently, over how to make peace, their leaders should start thinking more about the potential of synergy between their two peoples in many areas, as an asset for moving from confrontation to peace making. This book provides both general readers and specialists alike with successful approaches that can be replicated in both this tragic conflict and beyond."

Ambassador (ret.) Philip Wilcox, *Former U.S. Consul General, Jerusalem; Former President, Foundation for Middle East Peace, Washington, DC*

"Reading Norbert Goldfield's *Peace Building through Women's Health* was a surprisingly emotional experience for me. Initially I was filled with admiration for this group. For fifteen years they have held on to their belief that health work could contribute to peace. HATD has helped with diabetes, HIV, addictions, mental health, childhood accidents, and an astonishing array of health issues. They have used methods I admire – strengthening civil society organisations close to the communities involved, insisting on measuring the impact of their work. Their service to basic needs for health care in marginalized communities represents 'what is decent in an indecent world'.

Then I was flooded by sadness – the political vice tightening on the Palestinians is so appalling, the Israeli military prevents the most tentative of meetings across the divide. Humanitarianism is surely an inadequate stop-gap when the real need, political change, diminishes in probability. Norbert Goldfield himself acknowledges that 'resolution of the conflict...may not occur in my lifetime'.

Yet, HATD looks this full in the face and keeps on. I learned from and will hold on to their triple vision. In the short term, they know they are making a difference to hundreds of thousands of lives, contributing to healthier and stronger communities. In the medium term, they are strengthening leadership in civil society – a most valuable asset. In the long term, HATD hopes that these leaders, learning from the values and vision of the organization, will contribute to building peace. I salute them with all my heart!"

Joanna Santa Barbara, *coeditor of* Peace through Health: How Health Professionals Can Work for a Less Violent World, *has written extensively on peace through health. She is actively committed to the climate change movement and lives in New Zealand*

Peace Building through Women's Health

This book is an examination of the Israeli-Palestinian conflict through psychoanalytic, sociopsychological, and nationalistic lenses, highlighting the successes and the hurdles faced by one organization, Healing Across the Divides (HATD), in its mission to measurably improve health in marginalized populations of both Israelis and Palestinians.

Peace Building through Women's Health begins with a summary of the "peace building through health" field and a psychoanalytic, sociopsychological examination of the Israeli-Palestinian conflict. After a series of informative case studies, the book concludes with an analysis of how this organization has evolved its "peace building through health" approach over the fifteen years since its founding. Working with community groups, HATD has measurably improved the lives of more than 200,000 marginalized Israelis and Palestinians. In the process, it also improves the effectiveness of the community group grantees, by offering experienced management consulting and by requiring rigorous ongoing self-assessment on the part of the groups. HATD hopes that, in the long term, some of the community leaders it supports will be tomorrow's political leaders. As these leaders strengthen their own capabilities, they will be able to increasingly contribute to securing peace in one of the longest running conflicts in the world today.

Peace Building through Women's Health will be invaluable to public and mental health professionals interested in international health, peace and conflict studies, and conflict resolution.

Norbert Goldfield is founder and executive director of the American not-for-profit Healing Across the Divides. He is a practicing physician, editor of the *Journal of Ambulatory Care Management*, and has authored more than 50 articles and books. He believes that health professionals can and do play an important role in society beyond direct care.

Psychoanalytic Inquiry Book Series
JOSEPH D. LICHTENBERG
Series Editor

Like its counterpart, *Psychoanalytic Inquiry: A Topical Journal for Mental Health Professionals*, the Psychoanalytic Inquiry Book Series presents a diversity of subjects within a diversity of approaches to those subjects. Under the editorship of Joseph Lichtenberg, in collaboration with Melvin Bornstein and the editorial board of *Psychoanalytic Inquiry*, the volumes in this series strike a balance between research, theory, and clinical application. We are honored to have published the works of various innovators in psychoanalysis, including Frank Lachmann, James Fosshage, Robert Stolorow, Donna Orange, Louis Sander, Léon Wurmser, James Grotstein, Joseph Jones, Doris Brothers, Fredric Busch, and Joseph Lichtenberg, among others.

The series includes books and monographs on mainline psychoanalytic topics, such as sexuality, narcissism, trauma, homosexuality, jealousy, envy, and varied aspects of analytic process and technique. In our efforts to broaden the field of analytic interest, the series has incorporated and embraced innovative discoveries in infant research, self psychology, intersubjectivity, motivational systems, affects as process, responses to cancer, borderline states, contextualism, postmodernism, attachment research and theory, medication, and mentalization. As further investigations in psychoanalysis come to fruition, we seek to present them in readable, easily comprehensible writing.

After more than 25 years, the core vision of this series remains the investigation, analysis and discussion of developments on the cutting edge of the psychoanalytic field, inspired by a boundless spirit of inquiry. A full list of all the titles available in the *Psychoanalytic Inquiry* Book Series is available at https://www.routledge.com/Psychoanalytic-Inquiry-Book-Series/book-series/LEAPIBS.

Peace Building through Women's Health

Psychoanalytic, Sociopsychological, and Community Perspectives on the Israeli-Palestinian Conflict

Edited by
Norbert Goldfield

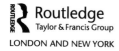
Routledge
Taylor & Francis Group

LONDON AND NEW YORK

First published 2021
by Routledge
2 Park Square, Milton Park, Abingdon, Oxon OX14 4RN

and by Routledge
605 Third Avenue, New York, NY 10158

Routledge is an imprint of the Taylor & Francis Group, an informa business

British Library Cataloguing-in-Publication Data
A catalogue record for this book is available from the British Library

Library of Congress Cataloging-in-Publication Data
Names: Goldfield, Norbert, 1952- editor.
Title: Peace building through women's health : psychoanalytic,
    sociopsychological, and community perspectives on the
    Israeli-Palestinian conflict / edited by Norbert Goldfield.
Description: Milton Park, Abingdon, Oxon ; New York, NY : Routledge, 2021.
    | Series: Psychoanalytic inquiry book series | Includes bibliographical
    references and index.
Identifiers: LCCN 2020048988 (print) | LCCN 2020048989 (ebook) | ISBN
    9780367757106 (hardback) | ISBN 9780367757113 (paperback) | ISBN
    9781003163657 (ebook)
Subjects: LCSH: Women--Health and hygiene--Middle East. | Public
    health--Political aspects. | Peace-building--Women.
Classification: LCC RA778 .P3143 2021 (print) | LCC RA778 (ebook) | DDC
    613/.042440956--dc23
LC record available at https://lccn.loc.gov/2020048988
LC ebook record available at https://lccn.loc.gov/2020048989

ISBN: 978-0-367-75710-6 (hbk)
ISBN: 978-0-367-75711-3 (pbk)
ISBN: 978-1-003-16365-7 (ebk)

Typeset in Times
by KnowledgeWorks Global Ltd.

Contents

Preface, acknowledgments, and organization of this book

Current events around the world make peace building more challenging than ever. Yet many health professionals continue to engage in activities that extend their Hippocratic Oath in the effort to have a positive, humanitarian impact on community, countrywide, regional, or even worldwide conflicts. This book will summarize the successes and highlight the hurdles of one organization, Healing Across the Divides (HATD), in its mission to measurably improve the health of marginalized populations of both Israelis and Palestinians. HATD aims to sow seeds of peace in the setting of an intractable peace-building challenge, the Israeli-Palestinian conflict. With the help of other contributors, I will place the work of Peace Building through Health (PtH) into wider theoretical frameworks.

This book is divided into three sections:

- an introductory section (two chapters) providing a summary of the field of PtH and background on aspects of the Israeli-Palestinian conflict;
- a case studies section (twelve chapters), consisting of detailed analyses of Healing Across the Divides (HATD)–funded initiatives;
- a final section (three chapters) describing how HATD has evolved its PtH approach since it was founded in 2004, together with a look at the future.

In the first chapter of the background section of this book, I introduce the concepts of PtH as developed since 1995. I connect these concepts to the Israeli-Palestinian conflict in general and, specifically, how staff at Healing Across the Divides have kept a focus on its mission while the ongoing conflict has led to a deterioration in the lives of

Palestinians living in the West Bank and Gaza. In the second chapter, I analyze the ongoing impact of psychic war trauma at the individual level for both Israelis and Palestinians. In this same chapter I then examine Israeli and Palestinian societal efforts to mitigate or, in fact, exacerbate this psychic trauma via group, particularly nationalistic, influences.

The case study section of the book presents eleven chapters on community-based groups that HATD has supported financially and organizationally since 2004. Each of these community-based groups has implemented initiatives over a period of three years of HATD support. Several of the chapters are co-authored with leaders of the organizations that we funded/worked with. A few of these initiatives have been so successful that governmental or quasi-governmental agencies have taken them over and implemented them on a wider scale. Some of these initiatives have unfolded, on the Palestinian side, under the twin linked challenges of increasing poverty and steadily encroaching occupation. In the last chapter of this section, Christine Seibold, using qualitative research, analyzes the impact HATD has had on the community-based groups it has supported since 2004.

In the final section of the book, I place the work of HATD in the context of recent writings on PtH that attempt to push the boundaries of what health professionals might be able to accomplish. Even as I pay tribute to the valiant efforts of health professionals to expand our potential impact on peace building through health, I explore why such efforts are extremely difficult to implement, especially in the setting of ongoing hostilities such as the Israeli-Palestinian conflict.

Over the past decade, we have seen an intensification in the Israeli-Palestinian conflict and an increase in attacks, physical and emotional, against health care professionals and health care institutions throughout the world. In this context, I include a chapter that deals with the challenges that Palestinian health care professionals face in their everyday struggle to provide care to Palestinians in the midst of one of the longest-running conflicts in the world today. These are one-sided challenges that the vast majority of Israeli heath care professionals do not face, are not fighting against, or even know they exist.

Keeping in mind realistic and effective PtH efforts in the Israeli-Palestinian context, the last chapter highlights future possibilities for Healing Across the Divides. This chapter briefly takes into account the impact of COVID-19 and other pandemics on PtH in the Israeli-Palestinian conflict. I outline a certainly incomplete list of those latter possibilities, as this is a new phenomenon. We can only hope that the positive impacts might prevail.

A note on terminology used in this book. While the country of Israel exists, the area that Palestinians and Israeli settlers reside in located beyond the 1967 border between Israel, Jordan, and Egypt is termed, in this book, Occupied Palestinian Territory or OPT. It is the term primarily employed by both the United Nations and the European Union. I use OPT here to indicate that the West Bank and Gaza are land under Israeli occupation and that negotiations are needed to resolve its status.

I take full responsibility for all the opinions and statements in this book. That said, I've benefited immeasurably from both the patient reading of the critical chapters of this book by Sandra Matthews, my wife, together with the expert editorial assistance of Lory Frankel. Daniel Bar-Tal commented on the sociopsychological section of chapter 2. Mordechai Kamel generously reviewed chapter 17 and made helpful suggestions. Lastly, thanks to Joe Lichtenberg for suggesting that I write this book in the first place and introducing me to the editors at Routledge-Taylor Francis.

This book could never have materialized without the amazing on-the-ground Healing Across the Divides representatives, its dedicated support staff, and the commitment of the HATD board of directors. Most important, though, are the community-based organization (CBO) grantees, with inspired leaders who thought of the ideas that they, in turn, implemented. It is to these CBOs, together with the HATD staff and the HATD board of directors, that this book is dedicated. Without these individuals—and yes, organizations are made up of individuals—there would be little likelihood of health improvement among the more than 200,000 lives that HATD has directly touched. Without the passion and hopes of all these individuals there would be no possibility of "healing across the divides."

Part I

Introduction and overview of the first fifteen years of Healing Across the Divides

Chapter I

Peace building through health

A review with specific attention to the Israeli-Palestinian conflict

Norbert Goldfield

This chapter will first define the term Peace through Health. I will then describe the tools that advocates of Peace Building through Health, the term I prefer, have developed. Finally, I will situate these in the evolution of activities that HATD has pursued since its founding in 2004.

Introduction

Peace through health was defined in 1995 by the World Health Organization (WHO) as follows: "When there is an underlying genuine thrust towards peace and reconciliation, Health can play a role as catalyst in the peace process."[1] Such initiatives were described in a recent United States Institute for Peace paper: "They are premised on the idea that cooperation among health professionals and health interventions in conflict zones can contribute not only to improved outcomes for populations who suffer from the impact of war, but also to building a lasting peace."[2] While developed only in the past thirty years, the idea of "Peace through Health" has already been realized through numerous efforts, starting with the Pan American Health Organization "Health as a Bridge to Peace" program, which included a vaccination scheme.[3] Its impact is reflected in the award of the Nobel Peace Prize to International Physicians for the Prevention of Nuclear War in 1985.[4]

This book explores a key question: What are the possible roles of health professionals in a setting of ongoing confrontation such as the Israeli-Palestinian conflict? Taking up such roles is challenging enough. Yet health professionals who accept this difficult task have been faced with the even greater challenge of attacks against them. These have spiraled out of control, particularly in the past decade, to the point that most combatants in wars going on in the world today do not perceive health professionals and their work as neutral and deserving of protection. These questions are addressed here through the lens of the organizations that Healing Across the Divides has funded and worked with.

I would like to state at the outset that I do not believe in the phrase "Peace through Health" as first articulated by the health professionals working at WHO in the early 1990s.[5] However, I completely agree with the concept that health professionals working in their professional capacity can contribute to peace building through health. Peace through health (or any other area) is a political process and requires the intervention of individuals/groups that have political standing (or "multi-track diplomacy," as it is called in the peace-building jargon). In contrast, peace building through health consists of creating "an environment that increases people's investment in peace and can reduce, if not relieve, tensions that contribute to conflict."[6] I founded Healing Across the Divides (hereafter HATD) in 2004 as an organization committed to peace building through health (hereafter PtH). HATD's mission is to measurably improve the health of marginalized Israelis and Palestinians via community-based interventions. Funding for HATD largely comes from individual donors together with partnerships with other foundations, nonprofits, and international agencies.

The tools of peace building through health

Researchers and policymakers have identified a number of specific tools that organizations have utilized to encourage PtH.[7] I will identify each of them separately, adding comments on their place in the Israeli-Palestinian conflict and in the operations of HATD.

"Strengthening of communities"

Among these "peace building through health" tools, HATD, in particular, has advocated the strengthening of communities. The objective behind the strengthening of communities and community-based organizations is not just to achieve health improvement for individuals but to accomplish this within a community-based framework. Communities are obviously made up of individuals. A PtH approach should measurably improve the inner strength, the confidence, and/or the resilience of individuals—all within a community context.

It is disparities between communities that lead to disparity in health between individuals. At the same time, an important aim of our approach to grant giving is to strengthen leadership of these organizations (see chapter 14). HATD believes that the strengthening of communities via health can encourage leaders of these communities who are open to it to engage with each other across divides. We have seen this happen across religious and political divides, such as between HATD-funded Israeli Arab and Jewish community-based groups that worked together to press the Israeli government on health care inequalities (see chapter 3). By supporting community-based groups, we aim to strengthen communities in several ways: to measurably improve the health of communities; improve the capacity of the community groups themselves; and, potentially of greatest political importance, increase the effectiveness of the leaders of these community groups.

"Communication of knowledge"

Communication of knowledge is another important "peace-building through health" tool. It is critical that this communication of knowledge occur in a setting of respect and a sense of equality between both parties. Thus, for example, some, but by no means all, Palestinian groups prefer not to receive training from Israeli groups, particularly if the Israeli group has not explicitly rejected the occupation of Palestinian territory. Using the approach specified above, HATD places significant value on training individuals and local organizations in research and evaluation techniques, which we believe are critical to the success of any community-based health intervention.

"Personalizing the enemy"

HATD, Physicians for Human Rights-Israel (PHR-Israel), and other organizations have endeavored to put a human face on suffering that takes a toll on both sides of the conflict. HATD has sponsored speaking tours in the United States of, for example, directors of HATD-funded initiatives aiming to improve diabetes care among Palestinians living in the Occupied Palestinian Territory (OPT), early detection of breast cancer among Orthodox Jewish women in Jerusalem, and health improvement among Arab or Palestinian women living in extremely impoverished conditions in the northern part of Israel.

"Construction of goals in common"

This approach offers a way to thread a needle between opposing sides on joint initiatives where there might be agreement. *Bridges*, a publication of the World Health Organization in the early 2000s that had both Israeli and Palestinian health professionals on its editorial board, represents one such effort (see chapter 15). It met with minimal success, as the journal never addressed the underlying political causes of, in particular, Palestinian health disparities—that is, the Israeli-Palestinian conflict. The articles themselves were somewhat generic, and few concrete joint projects seem to have emerged from this publication. It folded after only a few issues. While HATD does not demand that groups team up on projects, we bring willing organizations together for regular meetings. The meetings themselves do not constitute construction of goals in common, but groups that have attended these meetings have worked together across the divides.

"Medical and health professional clinical practice across the divides"

Health professionals in the Israeli-Palestinian conflict have always given of themselves, on an altruistic basis, to treat individuals suffering on the other side of the conflict. Israeli health professionals—both Jewish and non-Jewish—practice this on a daily basis, particularly in Israeli hospitals. Physicians for Human Rights-Israel, in particular, has engaged in this important "peace building through health" tool and has directly contributed to saving the lives of many Palestinians in the Occupied Palestinian Territory (OPT). Medical professionals can also extend solidarity merely by their presence and the use of their clinical skills—that is, by risking their own lives to treat people in war zones. Physicians for Human Rights-Israel has done this extensively. This organization was extremely supportive of Palestinians in Gaza and the West Bank during the most difficult and personally endangering period of the second intifada, which began in 2000. PHR-Israel continues to work in Gaza (see chapter 15). HATD professionals, members of our Scientific Advisory Board, and professional expert supporters have engaged in this work in both Israel and the OPT.

"Noncooperation and dissent"

This tool consists of medical personnel refusing to participate in what are considered unjust war campaigns of their governments. It has been adopted only minimally on the part of either Israeli or Palestinian health professionals in the Israeli-Palestinian conflict. As will be discussed in chapter 15, HATD does not engage in "noncooperation and dissent"; furthermore, it does not take political stances on the overarching Israeli-Palestinian conflict.

Healing Across the Divides: a personal, yet academic review of the years since our founding in 2004; milestones in the history of Healing Across the Divides

Some organizations and/or foundations interested in PtH directly deliver services (e.g., Doctors without Borders/Médecins sans Frontières and Physicians for Human Rights-Israel). Others focus on empowering individual social entrepreneurs (e.g., Ashoka). Still others, such as HATD, only fund and work with already existing local or community groups. As discussed in chapter 15 and in some of the case studies, we single out already established community groups for several reasons, partly in the expectation that we will be increasing the effectiveness of already strong leaders and also because we believe that in the Israeli-Palestinian conflict, peace, when it comes, will be driven locally by leaders of organizations respected in their own society (see chapter 17).

And yet, all new organizations begin with the singular impact of individuals. For Healing Across the Divides, four individuals were key to its foundation. They were present "at the creation" and encouraged its formation. The germ of HATD started well before its legal incorporation in 2004. In 1996, as part of a four-month sabbatical with my family, I practiced medicine in Israel and, for the first time, near Ramallah, OPT. One person in particular influenced my thinking and actions, leading to the development of HATD. This was Heidar Abu Ghosh, a colleague of mine with whom I worked in the village of Biddu, OPT, where I treated patients as an internist. At the time, he worked at the Palestinian Medical Relief Society, one of a number of non-governmental organizations (NGOs) that both directly deliver care and engage in political activity. Heidar, now a dear lifelong friend (I've been to the weddings of some of his children), was one of the first members of the HATD Board of Directors and has been an active supporter throughout HATD's history.

Drs. Zeev Wiener of Israel and Jumana Odeh Issawi from the Occupied Palestinian Territory were the speakers for a successful tour in 2004 sponsored by Physicians for Human Rights-USA on the impact of the Israeli-Palestinian conflict on health care.[8] Their presentations provided the immediate impetus for HATD's formation as an organizational entity. The leader of PHR-USA at the time was Len Rubenstein. He actively supported the formation of HATD both organizationally, via PHR-USA, and individually, as an original and long-serving member of the HATD Board of Directors. The mission of HATD at the time of its inception has basically remained the same ever since: to measurably improve the health of marginalized Israelis and Palestinians via community-based interventions. We do our work through already existing organizations in both Israel and the OPT. We bring them together and foster mutual work to the extent that they are willing.

What are the other milestones that I would like to highlight?

1 Very early on, we realized that one-year grants could not have the impact we hoped for. In one year, the sustainability and other outcomes of the initiatives that we aim at, as discussed in other chapters, cannot be accomplished. Within two years we switched our funding cycle to three-year grants, and that has been our funding approach ever since.

2 Despite our initial very small budget (less than $150,000), we quickly decided that we needed to hire a representative in Israel

and in the OPT. It is the local engagement between people on both sides of the Israeli-Palestinian conflict that is key to PtH. That political engagement must start "at home," and we have been successful in recruiting Israeli and Palestinian representatives who have worked well with each other.

3 We have always sought out partnerships with other organizations in which we share expenses, expertise, and decision making. We've jointly funded/provided technical advice to many initiatives undertaken by many groups (see the Appendix for a list of initiatives that HATD has funded). Partnerships with organizations such as the Jewish Federation of Cleveland and the United Nations High Commissioner for Refugees (UNHCR) allow us to learn from them, while we expose these organizations to our perspectives on the Israeli-Palestinian conflict.

4 We now have an annual Healing Across the Divides Study Tour. We have familiarized approximately one hundred American participants with the dual Israeli and Palestinian narratives so ever-present in this region, emphasizing the need to be open to both perspectives. An important part of HATD's political agenda is to engage Americans with the local political realities indirectly by exposing them to the health ramifications of this long-running conflict.

5 As a human being and a child of Holocaust survivors, I find the treatment by Israelis and the Israeli government of African Refugee Asylum Seekers (RAS) among the most personally painful aspects of a very challenging Israeli-Palestinian landscape. While our mission states that we work with "marginalized Israelis and Palestinians," the board, in another milestone, decided almost five years ago to expand the reach to groups working to measurably improve the lives of African RAS, all of whom are marginalized and virtually none of whom are considered Israeli. I am proud that for each of the last several years we have supported at least one Israeli community-based group working with RAS. I am also very proud that in supporting this work, we have often partnered with the UN High Commissioner for Refugees.

6 Another milestone, the gathering of all interested Israeli and Palestinian grantees twice a year, materialized several years ago on the recommendation of our Israeli and Palestinian representatives.

We meet in East Jerusalem, claimed by Palestinians as their capital and annexed by Israel. At the request of the grantees themselves, we don't publicize the events. I will never forget the look of amazement and happiness at the first meeting of two women, one from Yeroham in Southern Israel and another from Nablus in the northern West Bank, OPT—both of them working on similar gender-based issues. Yeroham and Nablus are about two hours from each other. The sad reality is that virtually no one from Yeroham would ever dream of going to Nablus, and vice versa. Healing Across the Divides made it happen.

Building on these milestones, HATD has impacted the lives of over 200,000 marginalized Israelis and Palestinians in both Israel and the OPT. Subsequent chapters in this book detail the successes and failures of the initiatives that HATD has funded. Learning from these opportunities for improvement, HATD staff, led by its board, will continue its mission of measurably improving the health of Israelis and Palestinians. Beyond this goal, we hope that some of the leaders of the organizations that we fund on both the Israeli and Palestinian sides of this conflict will become tomorrow's political leaders.

Appendix: HATD timetable

2004: Drs. Zeev Wiener of Israel and Jumana Odeh Issawi from the Occupied Palestinian Territory (OPT) were the speakers of a successful Physicians for Human Rights-USA–sponsored tour in the United States. Norbert Goldfield organized this tour with Len Rubenstein, JD, then director of PHR-USA. Healing Across the Divides is formed as a consequence of this study tour.

December 2004: HATD is incorporated. Two grants are given in the first year: a program focused on diabetics in the Ramallah area, OPT, via the Palestinian Medical Relief Society, and Physicians for Human Rights-Israel working with marginalized Russian Jews.

2006: HATD moved from a one-year grant cycle to a three-year grant cycle.

2006: Heidar Abu Ghosh is the first HATD grantee to visit the United States on an HATD-sponsored speaking tour. Along with HATD staff, Heidar visits/lectures at the State Department, Carnegie Endowment for International Peace, and Columbia University, among other institutions.

2006: Suheil Aqabnah, MD, is the first physician to come to the United States to supplement his clinical skills at the Mid-Hudson Family Practice Residency in Kingston, New York, as part of an HATD-sponsored initiative—an effort that lasted several years.

August 2008: Our first representative in Israel is hired.

2010: We form our first major partnership with another organization, Jewish Federation of Cleveland. We have worked for several years with the many dedicated Federation staff.

December 2015: We hire our first representative in the OPT.

2015: We fund our first program for African RAS in Tel Aviv, in partnership with the UNHCR, on the heels of a growing population fleeing war and poverty in their native homelands.

2015: The residents of Susiya, a Palestinian community benefiting from an HATD empowerment program for Palestinian mothers and families with Post-Traumatic Stress Disorder (PTSD), fight expulsion efforts and succeed in temporarily remaining on their land.

2015: Two Israeli *kupot* (managed care organizations) take over an HATD-funded initiative to increase mammography rates among ultra-Orthodox Jewish women.

2016: Sara Weinberger, a longtime HATD supporter, organizes the first Healing Across the Divides Study Tour.

2016: The first joint meeting of Israeli and Palestinian grantees is held. Up to then, Israeli groups met with each other on a regular basis, as did Palestinian groups.

2018: HATD's Grandmothers for Social Change in Israel program wins the prestigious 2018 Ministry of Welfare Knesset prize and an award from the Safe Kids Worldwide Childhood Injury Prevention Convention (PrevCon).

2020: HATD launches its first initiative in the besieged Gaza Strip via an organization, Diabetes Palestine, that works throughout the OPT.

Notes

1 World Health Organization, Health as a Potential Contribution to Peace. p. 5 Available at: https://www.who.int/hac/techguidance/hbp/HBP_WHO_learned_1990s.pdf. Accessed: June 3, 2020.

2 Rubenstein, L., (2010) Peace building through health among Israelis and Palestinians. *Peacebrief* United States Institute for Peace: p. 7, January 28. Available from: http://www.usip.org/files/resources/PB7%20Health.pdf. Accessed: October 28, 2019.

3 Quadros, C. and Epstein, D., (2002) Health as a bridge to peace: The PAHO Experience. *Lancet*, 360, pp: s24-s26. Available at https://www.thelancet.com/pdfs/journals/lancet/PIIS0140-6736(02)11808-3.pdf. Accessed: June 3, 2020.

4 Nobelprize.org. Accessed: June 4, 2020.

5 Peace through health was defined in 1995 by the WHO as follows: "Health is valued by everyone. It provides a basis for bringing people together to analyze, to discuss and to arrive at a consensus acceptable to all. The potential for using health as a mechanism for dialogue and even peace, has been demonstrated in situations of conflict" (WHO 1995). Put differently, in a recent United States Institute for Peace paper (Rubenstein 2010, p.1) such initiatives are described thus: "They are premised on the idea that cooperation among health professionals and health interventions in conflict zones can contribute not only to improved outcomes for populations who suffer from the impact of war, but also to building a lasting peace."

Rubenstein, L., (2010) Peace building through health among Israelis and Palestinians. *Peacebrief* United States Institute for Peace 7. Available from: http://www.usip.org/files/resources/PB7%20 Health.pdf. Accessed: October 28, 2019.

6 Rubenstein (2010) Ibid. Accessed: June 3, 2020.

7 MacQueen, G., & Santa-Barbara, J., (2000). Peace building through health initiatives. *BMJ (Clinical research ed.)*, *321*(7256), pp. 293-296. Available at: https://www.ncbi.nlm.nih.gov/pmc/articles/PMC1118283/pdf/293.pdf. Accessed: June 3, 2020.

Arya, Neil and Santa Barbara, Joanna. (2008) *Peace Through Health*. Virginia: Kumarian Press.

8 Physicians for Human Rights (2004) PHR announces tour on impact of Israeli-Palestinian crisis on health care. Available at: https://reliefweb.int/report/occupied-palestinian-territory/phr-announces-tour-impact-israeli-palestinian-crisis-health. Accessed: June 4, 2020.

Chapter 2

Psychic trauma and competing nationalisms in the Israeli-Palestinian conflict

Norbert Goldfield

Introduction

In this chapter, I address the antecedents of the Israeli-Palestinian conflict, focusing on two points of entry that are inextricably intertwined with each other: psychic (both individual and collective) trauma and competing nationalisms. Starting with psychic trauma, I look at the impact of the Israeli-Palestinian conflict on individuals, through psychoanalytic and socio-psychological lenses, as both these disciplines have significant published literature on this topic. In articulating these two perspectives on psychic trauma in the Israeli-Palestinian conflict, I am not specifying that one is right and the other is wrong. Instead, I am simply trying to describe, drawing on two disciplines, the considerable psychic trauma undergone by both sides, its effect on individual members of each society, and its consequent impact on the conflict.

In addition to significant psychic trauma, both Israeli and Palestinian societies have dueling nationalisms, which, in turn, influence how members of each society make sense of the conflict as they go about their daily activities. Nationalist sentiments communicated throughout both societies interact in a positive feedback loop with ongoing psychic trauma on both sides. That is, nationalist sentiments serve to strengthen psychic trauma and vice versa. This feedback loop makes resolution of the conflict even more difficult. It is exactly this feedback loop that Healing Across the Divides aims to engage with and, ideally, interrupt in its community-based interventions.

This chapter draws on extensive research investigating the impact of psychic trauma and nationalism on the perception of the "other." In looking at the effects of psychic trauma, I start with psychoanalytic perspectives and move on to the socio-psychological approach. I then discuss competing Israeli and Palestinian nationalisms with a focus on recent writings. If we are to engage in peace building through health, as Healing Across the Divides (HATD) has attempted to do since its founding in 2004, it is important to detail the psychic trauma and nationalist forces that PtH practitioners need to be aware of and understand in this part of the world. Such an awareness has guided our development philosophy and operations at HATD.

To illustrate the PtH challenges, I start with the following two historical vignettes. For the purposes of this chapter, in describing Israeli psychic trauma I distinguish between the Israeli Jewish population and the 20 percent of the population in Israel that is Palestinian or Arab (depending on how one defines oneself). While Palestinians living in Israel represent a significant percentage of the population (and may in fact hold the key to a peaceful resolution of the Israeli-Palestinian conflict), the dominant political, cultural, and even legal ethos in Israel is Israeli Jewish or, to be more specific, Zionist. Understandably, the psychic trauma experienced by the Palestinian population in Israel is completely different from that of the Israeli Jewish population.

A historical vignette highlighting one expulsion episode from the Nakba,[1] May 1948

Operation Broom. Interview with Palmach (part of the pre-Israel Jewish army) machine gunner Yerachmiel Kahanovich (YK) by filmmaker E. Sivan:

INTERVIEWER (I): Operation Broom, what is it? You simply stood in line and just …

YK: Yes, you march up to a village, you expel it, you gather round and have a bite to eat, and go on to the next village… .

I: But how?

YK: You mean by shooting?

I: How do you mean?

YK: We shot, we threw a grenade here and there. Just listen—there is one thing you have to understand: at first, once they heard shots, they took off with the intention of returning later.

I: But wait a sec, that was before May 15 (declaration of Israeli independence), that was before the Arab armies came.... Operation Broom then. How does it happen? Do you receive any information? Is it an organized campaign? ...

YK: Yigal Allon (at the time commander of the Palmach; eventually a general and acting Israeli Prime Minister) himself planned it. We moved from one place to the next.

I: What places? Can you tell me?

YK: We passed by Tiberias and moved from one village to the other, from one to the next.

I: So, you had orders to expel and clean up the villages?

YK: And then go home.[2]

A historical vignette highlighting one terrorist attack on Israeli Jews

Interview with Naftali Lau Levi, a child survivor of the Holocaust, by psychoanalyst Hanni Mann-Shalvi:

> Among other incidents, Naftali talks of how in April 1974, he found himself in the coast town of Maalot in Northern Israel, as terrorists took control of the local school....
>
> When the firing stopped, I ran ... to the building. Tens of boys and girls and several adults lay dead or injured on the floor, and several sat leaning against the wall screaming for help. The horrific scene sent me back thirty years to scenes I hadn't found release from since Auschwitz and Buchenwald. I stood there, helpless, feeling my legs collapsing beneath me. I hurried outside and sat on a curbstone....
>
> The Israeli warrior who can protect his own life and that of his family, is pitched against Naftali's father or grandfather, who couldn't do a thing. Unlike the Holocaust, the Israeli soldier is an answer to the helplessness of the school children and of Naftali, who once again faces the Holocaust. When Naftali read my interpretation of his emotions, he admitted wholeheartedly that I had hit the nail on the head.[3]

Why is it so difficult to resolve intractable conflicts peacefully? Psychoanalytic perspectives

According to Adib Jarrar, the late Palestinian psychoanalyst,

> "although we cannot draw symmetrical lines of 'truth' concerning the two peoples, we can say that they are both psychologically imprisoned for different reasons by their own narratives, memories, recollections, losses, pain, fears, anger, and perceptions of this conflict. For Palestinians in the Occupied Palestinian Territory (OPT), Arab countries and Palestinian Diaspora, the loss of Palestine, figuratively their own paradise, was both displacement and replacement by an invading hostile group; reversal of this traumatic reality is very difficult, and currently unattainable."[4]

As Dr. Jarrar frames it, Palestinians see the loss of the land in a very personal way as their displacement and replacement by an invading hostile group. Many Palestinians, such as Rashid Khalidi and others, would call the group "settler-colonials."[5] According to Jarrar, Palestinians hold the image of Palestine as both the lost Paradise and a caring and loving mother.[6] Palestinian and Arab poetry and novels refer to Palestine always with this kept image.[7] In an effort to maintain "this kept image," Palestinians in Israel, the OPT, and elsewhere have for many years marked the day of the Nakba, May 15, as an annual day of commemoration of the displacement of Palestinians that preceded and followed the Israeli Declaration of Independence in May 1948.

The Israeli process of erasing the memory of Palestinians' existence on their own land is not limited to places, properties, mosques, and churches of the living but has expanded to include the dead through the destruction of many Muslim cemeteries. As exemplified in the vignette above, researchers have documented how Israelis carried out a campaign of ethnic cleansing (or, from the Israeli Zionist perspective, national liberation). For example, in 1948, nearly 100,000 Bedouin lived in the Negev. Three years later, their numbers had dropped to 13,000.[8] In addition, many Israelis have attempted to this day to erase the memories of the Palestinians in their own country, on the land on which Palestinians have lived for millennia. Yet an

Israeli Jewish organization, Zochrot, founded in 2002, aims to promote acknowledgment and accountability for the ongoing injustices of the Nakba, the Palestinian catastrophe of 1948, and the reconceptualization of the Return as the imperative redress of the Nakba and a chance for a better life for all the country's inhabitants.[9]

In contrast, Israeli Jews, and most Jews throughout the world, see the establishment of the State of Israel on the exact same land as, in part, a religious or secular fulfillment of the Land of Israel, inhabited by Jews for thousands of years. The biblical idea of "the promised land," together with ongoing European anti-Semitism, gave birth to the Zionist movement at the end of the nineteenth century. However, to many Israeli Jews, the Holocaust, or Shoah, represents the primary event in the formation of Israel. The searing memory of this calamity had a profound impact on the Israeli body politic and how it looked out to the rest of the world. By the 1960s, every official diplomat visiting Israel was taken on a tour to the "Yad Vashem" Holocaust memorial, which was established in 1953. While tours to Yad Vashem are dutifully arranged and carried out, psychoanalysts have emphasized their own inability to fathom the emotional meanings of the Shoah.[10] As the historian and psychoanalyst Peter Loewenberg recently stated: "As a totality and a concept, the Shoah is incomprehensible.... When confronting the Shoah we are in the presence of a ferocity of hatred and a welter of primitive feelings in the perpetrators and impotent rage in the victims which in turn releases primitive feelings in ourselves that make understanding difficult if not virtually impossible."[11] The reality is that the Shoah, while incomprehensible, has had and continues to have an ongoing effect on the Israeli Jewish collective psyche, and psychoanalytic techniques can help to plumb its ramifications.[12]

The late Palestinian psychoanalyst George Awad and other psychoanalysts such as Henri Parens posited that the attitude toward the "other" (the way Israeli Jews view Palestinians, and vice versa) begins with anxiety before shifting into acceptance or fear, the latter leading to xenophobia.[13] Awad believed that accepting the "other" starts with anxiety, but that it can be grasped, albeit with difficulty, contributing added richness to one's life. Alternatively, many individuals decide that the "other" is dangerous and thus should be hated, dominated, or even destroyed. Paraphrasing Freud, Awad states that individuals use three defense mechanisms to shunt aside difficult experiences:

> The first is foreclosure or repudiation (Freud 1911) which refers to the capacity of the psyche to eject an experience from consciousness, but which is not then repressed and returns in the form of hallucinations or delusions. The second is negation, which Freud defined as saying that the "content of a repressed image or idea can make its way into consciousness, on condition that it is negative. The third is denial or disavowal which results in ego splitting which in turn is the ego's response to unbearable external realities.[14]

This presence of two peoples, both suffering from significant emotional traumas illuminated by psychoanalytic insights, in the same land to which both feel deeply connected, and both demanding to live in it constitutes the conundrum that has led to the ongoing Israeli-Palestinian conflict. I now turn to socio-psychological research for additional insights into these same emotional traumas.

Why is it so difficult to resolve intractable conflicts peacefully?[15] A socio-psychological perspective

Socio-psychological theory posits that an individual's thoughts and emotions are impacted by social factors or society. In the Israeli-Palestinian conflict, a societal culture of conflict serves to increase an individual's socio-psychological barriers to resolution of this long-standing conflict. This section will first highlight barriers at the societal level. I will then focus on an individual's cognitive, emotional, and motivational barriers. Later in this chapter, I will very briefly detail what psychoanalytic and socio-psychological perspectives, from a vast reservoir of research, offer in the way of interventions that could overcome aspects of this conflict. In very modest ways, Healing Across the Divides engages with these interventions as part of its grant-giving process.

Starting with barriers from a societal perspective, intractable conflicts such as the Israeli-Palestinian conflict, because of their lasting bloody severity, have a negative or even "imprinting" effect on most individual members of the entire society.[16] These effects can include severe and continuous negative psychological symptoms such as "chronic threat, stress, pain, uncertainty, exhaustion, suffering, grief, trauma, misery, and hardship."[17] Inevitably, people adapt to this stress in order to satisfy basic human needs. As part of this process, people develop a psychological infrastructure that enables them to cope with the challenges of intractable conflict. Thus, individual members of both Israeli and Palestinian societies, according to Daniel Bar-Tal, a leader in the socio-psychological study of conflicts, in general, and the Israeli-Palestinian conflict, in particular, have developed a set of

> functional beliefs, attitudes, emotions, values, motivations, norms, and practices. This repertoire provides a meaningful picture of the conflict situation, justifies the society's behavior, facilitates wide mobilization for participation in the conflict, effectively differentiates between the in-group and the rival, and enables the maintenance of a positive social identity and collective self-image. These elements of the socio-psychological repertoire, on both the individual and collective levels, gradually crystallize into a well-organized system of shared societal beliefs, attitudes, and emotions that penetrates into the society's institutions and communication channels and become part of its socio-psychological infrastructure.[18]

There are three interrelated parts, explained in more detail below, to this psychic infrastructure, according to Bar-Tal: "collective memories, an ethos of conflict, and collective emotional orientation."[19] These three parts, from a socio-psychological perspective, provide the necessary cognitive-emotional ingredients for members of society to continue with their lives. Paradoxically, these same ingredients also feed continuation of the conflict.

The first of the three parts of this psychic infrastructure—collective memories—describes, for all members of society, the outbreak of the conflict and its course in a systematic and meaningful manner. The second part, ethos of conflict, sets out the shared societal beliefs (such as the justness of one's goals, need for security, and sense of victimization) that become the central societal orientation to the conflict. Finally, just as individuals have emotions, societies can facilitate the development in individuals of a third part of the psychic infra-structure, a "collective emotional orientation." This state is a "result of particular societal conditions, common experiences, shared norms, and socialization in a society."[20] An example of these shared norms is participation in ceremonies that in turn become part of an individu-al's psychic infrastructure.

These three aspects of psychic infrastructure come to be embedded together and provide rationale for the continuation of the conflict. It is these three aspects (collective memory, ethos of conflict, and collective emotional orientation) that, from a socio-psychological perspective, dominate societies engaged in intractable conflicts. Once these three aspects become institutionalized and disseminated throughout society, they serve as the pillars of the "culture of con-flict." This culture of conflict "provides the dominant meaning about the present reality, about the past, and about future goals and serves as a guide for individual action."[21]

Tragically, it is these same aspects of psychic infrastructure that "freeze," using Bar-Tal's and other sociopsychologists' term, giving rise to a refusal to absorb any alternative knowledge that may facili-tate willingness to compromise and to resolve the conflict.[22] Because of this freezing, individuals ignore any information that might pro-vide a different narrative that could, in turn, result in an opening toward resolution of the conflict. Cognitive, motivational, emotional, and other processes complement each other to freeze, in particular, the psychic infrastructure's culture of conflict aspect. The next sec-tion defines and expands on these three components of freezing.

Cognitive processes, the first component of freezing, constitute the ways all individuals structure knowledge of themselves and of the world. Cognitive processes lead to freezing when the beliefs and narratives rigidly or unchangeably support the ongoing conflict. The second component of freezing is motivation. Individuals are motivated to have faith in the validity of their narrative of the "ethos of conflict and collective memory." If it meets their needs (these are "inherent needs that would be pursued in all circumstances, except total indi-vidual despair and apathy"[23]), then individuals are motivated to use cognitive strategies to reach conclusions consistent with these narra-tives. They are motivated to reject information that contradicts their conflict-supporting narratives and will readily accept information that supports their approach to the conflict. The emotional factor, consisting of "negative intergroup emotions," is the third component that affects freezing. Each emotion is tied to an assessment of the emotional stimulus that can emerge from societal beliefs in a culture of conflict.[24]

Societal beliefs in a culture of conflict are strongly related to negative emotions such as fear, hatred, and anger, widely shared by societal members. Fear is an important example of an emotion that may have such a negative impact that it induces a collective angst, meaning fear of possible group extinction. Furthermore, fear can result in an active search for certain types of information; a preference for information that highlights threats to the group the individual belongs to; an overestimation of the threat; and limits on the emergence of alternative strategies to cope with the conflict. Possibly of greatest concern, fear negatively affects cognitive processing, and it encourages a preference for "normal daily routines" and the avoidance of thinking outside the box. Fear, being a primary emotion that has a physiological evolutionary basis, overcomes hope in general and, specifically, the possibility of new ideas emerging that could resolve the intractable conflict.

In summary, freezing, triggered by numerous factors, is the dominant reason why societal beliefs in a culture of conflict function as socio-psychological barriers. These barriers lead members of society to select certain types of information that validate their held societal beliefs while ignoring and omitting contradictory information. Even when ambiguous or contradictory information is absorbed, it is cognitively integrated using bias and distortion.

The socio-psychological factors discussed above feed into societal barriers to the entry of information that could serve as a counter narrative to the need for the intractable conflict. Making the possibilities for resolution of the intractable conflict even more discouraging, political leaders and societal institutions, in order to stay in power, very often have their own stake in maintaining the conflict and thus also prevent alternative information that doesn't support a narrative of the need for an intractable conflict. According to Bar-Tal, political leaders and societal institutions favoring the continuation of the

conflict reinforce already existing perspectives of individual supporters using the following socio-psychological mechanisms:

> Examples of such mechanisms are (a) control of information that
> refers to selective dissemination of information about the conflict
> within the society by formal and informal societal institutions (e.g.,
> State Ministries, the Army, and the Media); (b) Censorship that refers
> to the prohibition on publication of information in various products
> (e.g., newspaper articles, cultural channels, and official publica-
> tions) that challenge the themes of the dominant conflict-supportive
> narratives; (c) discrediting of counter information that portrays
> information that supports counter-narratives and/or its sources
> (individuals or entities) as unreliable and as damaging to the inter-
> ests of the in-group; or (d) punishment that concerns use of sanctions
> against individuals who try to provide an alternative information.
> These mechanisms are constructed by the agents that are interested
> in the outbreak and continuation of the conflict.[25]

It is challenging for an organization like Healing Across the Divides
to modify the freezing that political leaders and/or societal institutions encourage. However, that is exactly what we try to do with the
partnerships that we form with other foundations, the successful
transfer of a small number of programs to either governmental or
quasi-governmental healthcare entities, and our attempts to engage
with and strengthen local community-based organizations in an
effort to maximize the success of their initiative.

It is also difficult to imagine a scenario in which a small nonprofit
group such as Healing Across the Divides (HATD) could possibly
affect, in particular, freezing of individuals. And yet it is exactly these
mechanisms (an ethos of conflict and collective emotional orientation) that peace building through health, via organizations such as
Healing Across the Divides, attempts to influence. Certainly, we do
not imagine ever doing this work at a national or societal level. But,
as discussed in the concluding chapter, our aim is to engage with both
Israeli and Palestinian community-based organizations and to reinforce or to increase the capacity of the remarkable leaders of these
groups. These organizations and these community leaders have the
potential to alter the freezing process described in this chapter.

Israeli and Palestinian nationalism

Throughout the world, but especially in the Middle East, nationalism does not necessarily correspond to having a nation or state. Neither Palestinians nor the Kurds have their own state. Although Armenians and Jews have states, that is a recent phenomenon. Importantly, Benedict Anderson, a foremost scholar of nationalism, highlights that "theorists of nationalism have often been perplexed if not irritated by the paradox ... of the objective modernity of nations to the historian's eye vs. their subjective antiquity in the eyes of nationalists."[26] As will be seen below, both Israeli and Palestinian historians and philosophers attest with absolute certainty to the fact that Palestinians and Jews have a national identity extending back for thousands of years.

Jews today have a homeland, and any Jew who wishes to move to Israel automatically becomes a citizen. Not only do Palestinians not have a homeland, but their population is divided in several ways, first between a global diaspora and the historic British mandate of Palestine that was in place from 1918 to 1948. Millions of Palestinians live outside the Arab Middle East. Then, within the geographic area covered by the British mandate, Palestinians are split between Israel, East Jerusalem, the West Bank, and Gaza. In addition, sizable Palestinian populations—in the millions—live in the Arab Middle East, in refugee camps (such as in Lebanon) or countries such as the Gulf States, where they typically cannot obtain citizenship.

These geographic facts on the ground impact Israeli and Palestinian nationalism. But they represent only one aspect of nationalism. There are, at least, three types of nationalism: First, territorial nationalism emphasizes the common territory and citizenship as the criteria for individuals' inclusion in the national group. The second type of nationalism, ethnic nationalism, posits that ethnic affiliation, regardless of location, is the criterion for inclusion within the national group. The third type of nationalism—the nationalism of the vulnerable, often economically disadvantaged—represents a revolt by this increasingly large percentage of a nation's population against global elites. Global elites often espouse a supranational world perspective. This third type of nationalism, which posits that the resolution of economic grievances lies in faith in the nation, finds a modest presence in Israeli nationalism, less so in Palestinian nationalism.

For the remainder of this section, I will focus on the recently published work of Palestinians Rashid Khalidi and Nur Masalha and Israelis Yael Tamir and Yoram Hazony. Nur Masalha begins his recently published book, *Palestine: A Four Thousand Year History*, thus: "First documented in the late Bronze Age, about 3200 years ago, the name Palestine (Arabic: Falastin), is the conventional name used between 450 BC to 1948 AD to describe a geographic region between the Mediterranean Sea and the Jordan River and various adjoining lands."[27] According to Rashid Khalidi, "Intellectuals, writers and politicians who were instrumental in the evolution of the first forms of Palestinian identity at the end of the last century and early in this century ... identified with the Ottoman Empire, their religion, Arabism, their homeland Palestine, their city or region, and their family, without feeling any contradiction, or sense of conflicting loyalties."[28]

Khalidi extensively documents that starting in the eighteenth century, Palestinian nationalism embodied a concern for the sacred nature of Jerusalem and its surrounding territory. The perception of the region's sacred, as opposed to political, essence was true for both Arab Christians and Muslims. This land was perceived to be under threat from external powers. For the past decades and still today, Palestinian identity has been intermixed with pan-Arabism, the Islamic *umma* (depending on its use, meaning "community," or even "nation"), and local, clan, or family loyalties. In the years before 1948, Palestinian identity was shaped by many external forces, including Zionists and also European powers that, for reasons related to Christianity and pure power plays, coveted the Middle East in anticipation of oil and land control. In response to Ottoman attempts to shut down the newspaper *Filastin* after the editor's attack on the Zionist movement, an editorial in May 1914 opined that "we are a nation [*umma*] threatened with disappearance in the face of this Zionist current in this Palestinian land."[29]

With the simultaneous expulsion of Palestinians and the defeat of Arab armies in 1948, nationalist Palestinian organizations formed, notably, the Palestine National Liberation Movement, known by its inverse acronym, Fatah, founded in the late 1950s. In 1964, the Palestine Liberation Organization was set up as an umbrella group, which Fatah later joined. The Popular Front for the Liberation of

Palestine was established in 1967. However, ideology, personality, and Arab power politics significantly diminished the unity of these nationalist Palestinian groups. The 1967 war that resulted in the total defeat of the Arab armies and a second expulsion of Palestinians only exacerbated the obstacles facing nationalist Palestinian groups. By 1970, "while a year earlier the fedayeen [Palestinian freedom fighters] had enjoyed the wholehearted support of almost all social strata, now only the refugee population and the poorer elements in the towns remained loyal to the resistance movement."[30] Five decades later, Palestinians are facing similar challenges as they try to develop a unified alternative to Israeli occupation of Palestinian territory. Hamas was formed in the 1980s. Palestinians and many others have invested much effort to resolve the ideological crisis and conflicts between Fatah and Hamas, with no success to date. A continuing existential crisis afflicts the Palestinians and their national movements, about which many have written.[31]

Continuing most recently with *The Virtue of Nationalism*, Yoram Hazony has expounded, in various publications, on the religious, philosophical, and territorial connections of the Jews and Israelis (after 1948) to the land of Israel. Hazony has written extensively about the philosophical and scriptural Hebrew antecedents of the State of Israel.[32] He directly links ancient Hebrew Scriptures and the nation of Israel. "Moses ... presents himself as legislating for Israel alone.... Hebrew Scripture maintains a permanent distinction between the national state sanctioned by Moses in Deuteronomy, which is to govern within prescribed borders; and the aspiration to teach God's word to the nations of the world."[33] While he, among many others, emphasizes these connections to the land of Israel, Hazony, echoing the vignette pertaining to the Holocaust quoted at the beginning of this chapter, points to the key event in the formation of Israel:

> For most Jews, Auschwitz has a very particular meaning. It was not Herzl's Zionist organization that persuaded nearly all Jews the world over that there could be no other way but to establish an independent Jewish state in our day. It was Auschwitz, and the deaths of six million Jews at the hands of the Germans and their sympathizers that accomplished this.[34]

In his writings, Hazony has also explored the political thought of many leading Jewish intellectuals who opposed the creation of Israel prior to its founding in 1948, including Martin Buber, Gershom Scholem, Albert Einstein, and Hannah Arendt. Their opposition highlights the ambivalence of many Jewish intellectuals, an attitude that persists to this day, about the national identity of Israeli Jews, diaspora Jews, and "Israeli-ness" (or Israeli nationalism). In some ways akin to Khalidi's discussion of Palestinian allegiances to family, a Palestinian nation, and Arab consciousness, many Jews throughout the world, including those in Israel, maintain multiple allegiances. Ten percent of all Israeli Jews live in the United States. Many American Jews and Jews from other countries, in addition, have made "aliyah," or immigrated to Israel. Other American Jews have an ineradicable commitment to the United States but at the same time feel that their fate is inextricably intertwined with the State of Israel as a homeland for the Jews.[35]

Yael Tamir, in her just published book, *Why Nationalism*, underlines the need for citizens of any country to view "the political framework as their own." She also points out, quoting Roger Brown, that conflict between different ethnic groups is a "sturdy three legged stool" composed of individual psychological makeup (as discussed earlier in this chapter), the ineradicable tendency of people to gather in ethnic groups, or the "nationalist impulse," and inequitable distribution of resources.[36] Tamir believes that we should spend less time "waging a war against the human tendency to gather in groups … and more on joining forces to combat social inequality and injustice."[37] While a salutary statement, Tamir, unfortunately, has little to say about two ethnic groups that want the same land with, up to now, one clear victor, while the other has not been willing to either give up its ethnic identity or simply leave the land.

Paralleling the fundamental quandary facing Palestinian nationalism, significant, though different, problems confront Israeli nationalism. For both nationalisms, according to Tamir, "one challenge lies in the past, the other in the present. One is the possession in common of a rich legacy of memories; the other is present-day consent, a desire to live together, a will to perpetuate the value of the heritage that one has received in an undivided form."[38] The issue is how the state/nation tries to shape this rich legacy of memories in an effort to maximize consent among its citizens. These memories also very much underlie our individual psychoanalytic and socio-psychological constructs discussed above. The nation, the state, and political elites shape these constructs, whether through five minutes of standing at attention as part of Holocaust Remembrance Day or the Palestinian celebration of martyrs on the day of the Nakba.

On the one hand, both Israeli and Palestinian nationalisms boast an extensive legacy of memories. Jews certainly manifest the desire to live with each other; the same desire to live together applies to Palestinians. On the other hand, the present-day national consent and the perpetuation of the value of a heritage in undivided form hold ambivalence for both Israelis (judging by the need for numerous recent elections to form a government) and Palestinians (judging from the lack of reconciliation between Hamas and Fatah). In the short term, at present, both Israelis and Palestinians display little tolerance for deviations from the value of a common heritage—or, using a socio-psychological perspective, we could say there is a "culture of conflict."[39] Possibly, in the long term, the challenges to national consent and to the value of the heritage could lay the groundwork for a compromise between Israelis and Palestinians. The opportunities for such a compromise, which recognizes the current unequal nature of the relationship between Israelis and Palestinians, are discussed further in the next section and in chapter 17.

Psychoanalytic and sociopsychological-based conflict-mitigating interventions

According to psychoanalyst Salman Akhtar, "since terrorism is a multiply determined phenomenon, the 'treatment' of dehumanization associated with it should approach the issue from multiple vantage-points that, in the end form a harmonious gestalt of purpose."[40] Specifically, Dr. Akhtar advocates interventions that enhance the confidence and/or engagement of the "oppressed" people. He pointedly reminds us that hatred is rooted in hurt and shame, and he emphasizes the importance of decreasing the "rage" the "oppressed people" feel and of developing interventions that build "empathy toward their oppressors," especially education that humanizes "the other."[41] In an essay appearing in the same volume as Dr. Akhtar's essay, *Violence or Dialogue: Psychoanalytic Insights on Terror and Terrorism*, the psychoanalyst

Dr. George Awad stresses that psychoanalytic insights are critical for "humanizing the other, rather than contributing to further polarization, misunderstanding and hatred."[42]

There exists an extensive literature of socio-psychological interventions, most done on a research basis, aimed at mitigating the Israeli-Palestinian "culture of conflict."[43] These interventions, focused on impacting cognitive, motivational, and/or emotional factors, can have the net result of unfreezing the "culture of conflict" described above. Thus, for example, in an experiment dealing with cognitive factors, when both Jewish and Palestinian citizens of Israel recognized their "naïve realism" ("The conviction that one's own views are objective and unbiased, whereas the other's views are biased by ideology, self-interest, and irrationality"), they were more open to new information presenting their opponents' perspective, even if this information did not mesh with their own long-held beliefs.[44] In another example, Bar-Tal noted that "Čehajić-Clancy and colleagues found that affirming a positive aspect of the self can increase one's willingness to acknowledge in-group responsibility for wrongdoing against others, countering the motivation to maintain a positive view of the in-group at all costs."[45] Many of these research interventions could form the basis of large-scale interventions that could lead, one day, to greater equality and mutual respect between Israelis and Palestinians.

Conclusions

This chapter provides a brief survey of the extensive literature on both the psychic trauma that has preceded and continues to nurture the Israeli-Palestinian conflict, together with the impact of Israeli and Palestinian nationalisms on it. According to sociopsychologists, several societal factors serve to strengthen continuation of this conflict. First and foremost, as stated by Daniel Bar-Tal, "societies in conflict develop conflict-supporting ideologies, consisting of societal beliefs that serve as building blocks of narratives about the past (collective memory) and the present (ethos of conflict)."[46] Today, unfortunately, political leaders in both Israel and the OPT, but particularly in Israel, strengthen these conflict-supporting ideologies by influencing the type of information that they or the governments they lead present to the public. Israeli political leadership influences information for the purpose of increasing the occupation and support for the annexation of Palestinian land in the OPT. Both sides carefully monitor non-governmental organizations and deal harshly with individuals that have a different point of view on conflict-supporting ideologies.[47]

To offer a differing but complementary perspective, this chapter has also examined the same socio-psychological barriers from a psychoanalytic perspective. Both psychoanalytic and socio-psychological research provides us with ample understanding of why the Israeli-Palestinian conflict persists with no end in sight. Finally, this chapter has summarized, via a look at two Israeli and two Palestinian philosophers and historians, the extensive work that researchers have produced on both Israeli and Palestinian nationalism. In the absence of leaders on either side who can "heal across the divides," it is Israeli and Palestinian nationalisms that supply the key ingredient that up to now only continues to exacerbate the "culture of conflict" in Israel and the Occupied Palestinian Territory (OPT).

An ethnic narrative that ties individuals to their larger group underlies each and every nationalist movement. If a nationalist movement is to foster peace building, the accommodation of the place of the "other's narrative" is key. Psychoanalytic and/or socio-psychological interventions, such as those referenced above, that could help resolve the Israeli-Palestinian conflict must in a modest way lead to acknowledgment of the validity of the "other's narrative." As stated by the psychoanalyst George Awad: "These [Israeli-Palestinian] narratives are as compelling and as 'truthful' as any other narratives. They do not negate the legitimacy of other narratives, but they need to be heard as representing ignored narratives. Only when both sides accept the legitimacy of the other's narrative can true communication and negotiation start."[48]

I contend that accepting the legitimacy of the other's narrative can come only when both sides feel strong, not just about their own legitimate narrative but also their own organizational, communal, and societal strengths. That is why Healing Across the Divides aims to strengthen the work of leaders within community-based organizations (CBOs) and the overall effectiveness of the CBOs that we fund. The next section of this book provides the eleven case studies of interventions undertaken with grants from HATD, with a concluding chapter on the impact of HATD on the leadership of the NGOs that we have funded and worked with.

Notes

1 "May 14 marks the 70th anniversary of Israel's founding; May 15 is a day Palestinians know as their *Nakba*, or 'catastrophe,' the traumatic expulsion of hundreds of thousands of Palestinians from their homes in 1948 by Israelis. This event both defined their future of statelessness and occupation, and now forms the basis for their distinct national identity. Many of the chief consequences of the *Nakba* including the displacement of most Palestinians from their ancestral lands and ongoing statelessness, remain unresolved to this day." Hussein, I. (2018) A 'Catastrophe' That Defines Palestinian Identity: For the people of Palestine, the trauma of 70 years ago never ended. *The Atlantic.* May 2018. Available at: https://www.theatlantic.com/international/archive/2018/05/the-meaning-of-nakba-israel-palestine-1948-gaza/560294/.

2 Transcribed testimony of Yerachmiel Kahanovich. Sivan E. (2012) *Towards a Common Archive – Video Testimonies of Zionist Fighters in 1948.* Available at: https://www.youtube.com/watch?v=lDEiUY8mW0Y. as quoted In Ross A. (2019). *Stone Men: The Palestinians who Built Israel.* New York: Vero; pp: 13–14.

3 Mann-Shalvi, H. (2016) *From Ultrasound to Army: The Unconscious Trajectories of Masculinity in Israel.* London: Karnac pp: 140–141.

4 Jarrar, A. (2010) Palestinian Suffering: Some Personal, Historical, and Psychoanalytic Reflections, *Int. J. Appl. Psychoanal. Studies* 7(3) pp: 197–208.

5 Khalidi, R. (2020). *The Hundred Years' War on Palestine: A History of Settle Colonialism and Resistance 1917-2017.* New York: Metropolitan Books.

6 Jarrar, A. (2010) Palestinian Suffering: Some Personal, Historical, and Psychoanalytic Reflections, *Int. J. Appl. Psychoanal. Studies* 7(3) p. 197.

7 Jarrar I. p. 197.

8 Shezaf, H. (2019) Burying the Nakba: How Israel Systematically Hides Evidence of 1948 Expulsion of Arabs *Haaretz* Available at: https://www.haaretz.com/israel-news/.premium.MAGAZINE-how-israel-systematically-hides-evidence-of-1948-expulsion-of-arabs-1.7435103. Accessed: May 2, 2020.

9 Our Vision (2002). *Zochrot* website Available at: https://www.zochrot.org/en/content/17 Accessed: May 9, 2020.

10 Brenner, I. (Ed) (2020) *The Handbook of Psychoanalytic Holocaust Studies.* New York: Routledge.

11 Loewenberg, P. (2020) Freud, Max Weber and the Shoah In Brenner I. (Ed.) *The Handbook of Psychoanalytic Holocaust Studies.* New York: Routledge. p. 18.

12 Brenner, I. (Ed) (2020) *The Handbook of Psychoanalytic Holocaust Studies.* New York: Routledge. 1st edition.

13 Parens, H. (1999) Toward the Prevention of Prejudice. In: Brescia MRF and Lemlif J. At the Threshold of the Millenium: A Selection of the Proceeding of the Conference. Peru: Sidea.

14 Awad, G. (2007) Prejudice between Israelis and Palestinians. In: Parent, H., Mahfouz, A., Twemlow, S., Scharff, D., *The Future of Prejudice: Psychoanalysis and the Prevention of Prejudice.* Plymouth: Rowan and Littlefield p. 187.

15 Title taken from Bar-Tal, D., Halperin, E., and Pliskin, R., (2015) Why Is It So Difficult to Resolve Intractable Conflicts Peacefully? A Sociopsychological Explanation In M. Galluccio (Ed.), *Handbook of International Negotiation: Interpersonal, Intercultural, and Diplomatic Perspectives.* Switzerland: Springer. See also Bar-Tal, D. (2013). *Intractable conflicts: Socio-psychological foundations and dynamics.* Cambridge: Cambridge University Press.

16 Bar-Tal, D., Halperin, E., and Pliskin, R., (2015) Why Is It So Difficult to Resolve Intractable Conflicts Peacefully? A Sociopsychological Explanation In M. Galluccio (Ed.), *Handbook of International Negotiation: Interpersonal,*

Intercultural, and Diplomatic Perspectives. Switzerland: Springer. p.74-see also Bar-Tal, D., & Halperin, E. (2011). Socio-psychological barriers to conflict resolution. In D., Bar-Tal (Ed.), *Intergroup conflicts and their resolution: A social psychological perspective* (pp. 217–240). New York: Psychology Press.

17 Ibid p. 74.

18 Ibid p. 74.

19 Ibid p. 74.

20 Bar-Tal, D; Halperin, E; and de Rivera, J. (2007) Collective Emotions in Conflict Situations: Societal Implications. *Journal of Social Issues*, Vol. 63, No. 2, pp. 442.

21 Bar-Tal, D., Halperin, E., and Pliskin, R., (2015) Why Is It So Difficult to Resolve Intractable Conflicts Peacefully? A Sociopsychological Explanation In M. Galluccio (Ed.), *Handbook of International Negotiation: Interpersonal, Intercultural, and Diplomatic Perspectives.* Switzerland: Springer. p. 75.

22 Ibid. p. 81.

23 Burton, JW. (2001) Conflict Prevention as a Political System. *The International Journal of Peace Studies.* (6)1 Available at: http://www.gmu.edu/programs/icar/ijps/vol6_1/Burton2.htm.

24 Roseman, J. (2013) Appraisal in the Emotion System: Coherence in Strategies for Coping. *Emotion Review Vol 5: no 2. 141–149.*

25 Bar–Tal, D., Halperin, E., and Pliskin, R., (2015) Why Is It So Difficult to Resolve Intractable Conflicts Peacefully? A Sociopsychological Explanation In M. Galluccio (Ed.), *Handbook of International Negotiation: Interpersonal, Intercultural, and Diplomatic Perspectives.* Switzerland: Springer. paraphrased on pages 77-29.

26 Anderson, B. (2006) *Imagined Communities: Reflections on the Origin and Spread of Nationalism.* U.K.: Verso, p.5.

27 Masalha, N. (2018) *Palestine: A Four Thousand Year History.* London: Zed Books, p. 1.

28 Khalidi, R. (1997) *Palestinian Identity: The Construction of Modern National Consciousness;* New York: Columbia University Press. P 19.

29 Ibid. p. 155.

30 Sharabi, H. (1971). Palestine Resistance: Crisis and Reassessment. *Middle East Newsletter* (Beirut) in Quandt, WB; Jabber F; Lesch AM. (1973) *The Politics of Palestinian Nationalism.* Berkeley: Univ California Press. P 199.

31 Khalidi, R (2020). *The Hundred Years' War on Palestine: A History of Settler Colonialism and Resistance 1917–2017.* New York: Metropolitan Books. See especially last chapter.

32 Hazony, Y (2012) *The Philosophy of Hebrew Scripture.* New York: Columbia University Press.

33 Hazony, Y. (2018) *The Virtue of Nationalism* New York: Basic Books, p. 225.

34 Hazony, Y. (2018) *The Virtue of Nationalism* New York: Basic Books, p. 202.

35 Graizbord, D. (2020). *The New Zionists: Young American Jews, Jewish National Identity, and Israel.* New York: Lexington Books.

36 Brown, R. (1986) *Social Psychology* New York: Free Press p 533 in Tamir, Y. (2019) *Why Nationalism.* New Jersey: Princeton University Press, p. 50.

37 Tamir, Y. (2019) *Why Nationalism.* New Jersey: Princeton University Press, p. 51.

38 Renan, E. What is a Nation, in Babha, HK (ed) 1990 *Nation and Narration* London: Routledge as quoted in Tamir *Why Nationalism?*, p. 56.

39 Litman, S. (2020) After Losing Hope for Change, Top Left-wing Activists and Scholars Leave Israel Behind. *Haaretz* Available at https://www.haaretz.com/israel-news/.premium.MAGAZINE-losing-hope-for-change-top-left-wing-activists-and-scholars-leave-israel-behind-1.8864499 Accessed: June 3, 2020.

40   Akhtar, S. (2003). Dehumanization: origins, manifestations and remedies in: Varvin S and Volkan V (eds). *Violence or Dialogue: Psychoanalytic insights on Terror and Terrorism* 1st ed London: International Psychoanalytic Association p. 143.

41   Akhtar, S. (2003). Dehumanization: origins, manifestations and remedies in: Varvin S and Volkan V (eds). *Violence or Dialogue: Psychoanalytic insights on Terror and Terrorism* 1st ed London: International Psychoanalytic Association p 143-145. And for more information on the impact of education please see Sherwood, H. (2013). Israeli and Palestinian Textbooks Omit Borders. *The Guardian* available at https://www.theguardian.com/world/2013/feb/04/israeli-palestinian-textbooks-borders. Accessed: June 3, 2020.

42   Awad, G. (2003). The mind and perceptions of the "others" in: Varvan S and Volkan V (eds). *Violence or Dialogue: Psychoanalytic insights on Terror and Terrorism* 1st ed London: International Psychoanalytic Association p. 155.

43   For more information please see: Sharvit, K. and Halperin, E. (2015) *A Social Psychology Perspective on The Israeli- Palestinian Conflict Celebrating the Legacy of Daniel Bar-Tal, Vol I.* New York: Springer Verlag. And Sharvit, K. and Halperin, E. (2016) *A Social Psychology Perspective on The Israeli-Palestinian Conflict Celebrating the Legacy of Daniel Bar-Tal, Vol II.* New York: Springer Verlag.

44   Nasie, M., Bar-Tal, D., Pliskin, R., Nahhas, E., & Halperin, E. (2014). Overcoming the barrier of narrative adherence in conflicts through awareness of the psychological bias of naïve realism. *Personality and Social Psychology Bulletin*, 40:11. p. 1543.

45   Bar-Tal, D., Halperin, E., and Pliskin, R., (2015) Why Is It So Difficult to Resolve Intractable Conflicts Peacefully? A Sociopsychological Explanation In M. Galluccio (Ed.), *Handbook of International Negotiation: Interpersonal, Intercultural, and Diplomatic Perspectives.* Switzerland: Springer, p. 89.

46   Ibid, p. 86.

47   Palestine: No Letup in Arbitrary Arrests, Torture. Palestinian Authority, Hamas Muzzle Critics, Opponents. *Human Rights Watch*. Available at https://www.hrw.org/news/2019/05/29/palestine-no-letup-arbitrary-arrests-torture. Accessed: June 3, 2020.
       Litman, S. (2020) After Losing Hope for Change, Top Left-wing Activists and Scholars Leave Israel Behind. *Haaretz* Available at https://www.haaretz.com/israel-news/.premium.MAGAZINE-losing-hope-for-change-top-left-wing-activists-and-scholars-leave-israel-behind-1.8864499 Accessed: June 3, 2020.

48   Awad, G. (2003). The mind and perceptions of the "others" in: Varvan S and Volkan V (Eds). *Violence or Dialogue: Psychoanalytic insights on Terror and Terrorism* 1st ed London: International Psychoanalytic Association, p. 175.

Part II

Case studies

Chapter 3

Ahli Balatah Al-Balad Club

Impacting diabetes control with a focus on chronic disease self-management

Norbert Goldfield and Mohammed Khatib

Introduction

HATD has spent more time and resources on community interventions pertaining to diabetes than any other health issue. In total, we have funded six different community groups—four in the Occupied Palestinian Territory (OPT) and two in Israel. One of the two Israeli groups was an Ethiopian Jewish community group, while the other was a Palestinian community organization serving Palestinians living in Israel. The six groups, together with the location of their headquarters, appear here in the order of their implementation: the Palestinian Medical Relief Society, or PMRS (Ramallah, OPT); the Galilee Society (Tamra, Israel); Tene Briut (Hadera, Israel); Family Defense Society, or FDS (Nablus, OPT); Caritas (East Jerusalem, OPT); Ahli Balatah Al-Balad Club, or ABBC (Nablus, OPT); and Diabetes Palestine (East Jerusalem and Gaza, OPT).

This introduction will summarize the chapter and then call attention to worldwide trends in diabetes through the lens of socioeconomic disparities. In the next section, we concentrate on community-based prevention and treatment of diabetes placed within the context of the Israeli-Palestinian conflict. It is followed by the results of the first three interventions—some of which worked and some that failed, at least in terms of programmatic results. We will then review the rationale and implementation of the three most recent interventions. These last three community-based interventions used a relatively new evidenced-based approach that has been translated and validated in Arabic: the Chronic Disease Self-Management Program, or CDSMP, developed at Stanford University.[1] We will both highlight results of the CDSMP initiatives and point to the political (in its broad sense) implications of an intervention such as the CDSMP. Other than extensive documentation of the positive impact of the CDSMP, this program has some intangible organizational benefits relevant for peace building through health (PtH). The concrete nature of the CDSMP (i.e., there is a very detailed manual with a defined mode of instruction) can facilitate communication between community-based groups about their interventions. In addition, the tangible nature of the CDSMP demonstrates that community-based groups have something to offer other, more powerful, organizations, such as Ministries of Health.

Before the discovery of insulin in 1921, diabetes was an epidemic. Elliot P. Joslin, one of the early researchers into diabetes, documented almost one hundred years ago the ravages it caused:

> In a country town in New England ... on its peaceful, elm-lined Main Street, there once stood three houses, side by side, as commodious and attractive as any in the village. In these three houses lived in succession four women and three men—heads of families—and of this number, all but one has subsequently succumbed to diabetes.... Although six of the seven persons dwelling in these adjoining houses died from a single complaint, no one spoke of an epidemic. Contrast the activities of the local and state boards of health if these deaths had occurred from scarlet fever, typhoid fever or tuberculosis. Consider the measure which would have been adopted to discover the source of the outbreak and to prevent a recurrence. Because the disease was diabetes, and because the deaths occurred over a considerable interval of time, the fatalities passed unnoticed.[2]

Diabetes is still an epidemic, but it has the added layer of pronounced socioeconomic disparities. I would like to highlight three points pertaining to overall changes in worldwide patterns of diabetes and socioeconomic disparities in health. First, while the worldwide prevalence has dramatically increased in just the last twenty-five years (from 1973–99, it increased by a multiple of 2.3 in the United States; from 1978–96, by 3.9 in Egypt), the burden of illness has disproportionately fallen on the poor and disadvantaged.[3] Second, there is a significant bidirectional relationship between mental health disorders and diabetes. Individuals with co-morbid chronic illnesses such as schizophrenia and diabetes have worse outcomes (earlier death and hospitalizations) and more costly treatments.[4] Third, and for me, most dramatically, recent research has demonstrated not only a relationship between stress, in general, diabetes, and poverty but also that these negative experiences of stress, especially if they occur in childhood, can impact the genes of children in their lives as well as their offspring. In more technical terminology: "chronic psychosocial stressors and related emotional states lead to dysfunctional mitochondria, which in turn contribute to stress pathophysiology via multiple mechanisms including changes in gene expression and the epigenome, alterations of brain structure and functions, abnormal stress reactivity, inflammation, and by promoting cellular aging."[5]

Socioeconomic disparities in diabetes with a focus on the Israeli-Palestinian conflict

Just as in other First World countries, there are significant socioeconomic disparities documented in Israel relative to non-communicable chronic diseases (NCDs). Diabetes, the focus of this chapter, is significantly higher among Palestinians living in Israel in comparison with Jews.[6] Life expectancy among Palestinians living in Israel is lower compared with that of Jews.[7] This gap is widening. In addition, significant differences in health care utilization exists; for example, there are higher rates of hospitalizations among Palestinians living in Israel.[8] It is particularly important to note the difference in rates of smoking: 45% of Palestinian men living in Israel versus 22% of Jewish men and 15% of Jewish women.[9]

For Palestinians living in the OPT, prediabetes or metabolic syndrome in some parts of the OPT, according to projections, has reached epidemic proportions.[10] In the Gaza Strip, a recent epidemiological survey documented that 41% of adults over the age of 25 had pre-diabetes, also called metabolic syndrome.[11]

A case study recently reported the situation confronting Palestinian diabetics in the OPT:

"We live a life of poverty," Abu Abdullah, a man in his late fifties, told Al Jazeera. Abu Abdullah said he moved three decades ago, after the Israeli army forced him off his land in the South Hebron Hills. Since the move, it has been hard for him to earn enough money to provide for his wife and seven children. His story is far from unique, as Israel controls nearly all aspects of Palestinian economic life. Palestinian arable land occupied by Israel for military and settler use amounts to two-thirds of the West Bank, leaving Palestinian unemployment rates among the highest in the world. "Poverty and unemployment is directly linked to inactivity and a poor diet. That is a recipe for diabetes," said Ahmad Abu al-Halaweh, who manages the mobile clinic and serves as director of the Diabetes Care Center at the Augusta Victoria Hospital in occupied East Jerusalem. An estimated 15 percent of Palestinians have been officially recorded as suffering from diabetes, compared with a global average of 9 percent. But Abu al-Halaweh believes the real number in Palestine is higher—more than 20 percent. The Israeli occupation has exacerbated the diabetes crisis in a number of ways, "especially the psychological stress that comes from it," Abu al-Halaweh added. "People in Gaza or Palestinian refugees suffer from an even poorer diet," he said, noting that one-third of Palestinians are considered to be short of food.[12]

Lastly, in 2011, there were 125,000 Ethiopian Jews in Israel, making up about 2% of the population. Ethiopian Jews began arriving in Israel in large numbers in the 1980s and 1990s. Studies in Israel have revealed that Ethiopian-Israeli diabetics use fewer health services than their counterparts and do not undergo routine follow-up tests.[13] Only 48% of Ethiopian patients say they understand medical staff, compared with 92% of others surveyed. As many as 82% of Ethiopian patients understand little or nothing of the pharmacists' instructions, compared with 20% of others; and 55% state they understand little or nothing of the advice given by dieticians.[14] Finally, and most importantly, diabetes was virtually unheard of in Ethiopia among Ethiopian Jews. The prevalence of diabetes for Ethiopian Jews in Israel ranges up to 20%.[15]

Results of the first three interventions: the implementing institutions

The Palestinian Medical Relief Society/PMRS (formerly, Union of Palestinian Medical Relief Committees), a grassroots, community-based Palestinian health organization, was founded in 1979 by a group of Palestinian doctors and health professionals seeking to fill the gap in primary health care services in rural areas of Palestine during the period of Israeli military occupation. It is nonprofit, voluntary, and one of the largest health nongovernmental organizations (NGOs) in Palestine. Notably, one of the founders and its current CEO is Mustafa Barghouthi, a physician, who ran second against President Mahmoud Abbas in the last Palestinian elections held in the OPT in 2005 (see chapter 15 for an in-depth examination of the roles of health professionals in politics).[16]

The Galilee Society: The Arab National Society for Health, Research and Services is a Palestinian Arab, community-wide NGO located in Israel, established by four health care professionals in 1981. Its overriding goal is to achieve equitable health, environmental, and socioeconomic conditions and to increase opportunities for development for Palestinian Arabs inside Israel, both as individual citizens and as a national minority living in their homeland. The Galilee Society consists of four departments through which it carries out its work: the Institute for Applied Research, Rikaz Center for Social Research, the Health Rights Center, and the Environmental Justice Center.

Tene Briut is a national Israeli community-based outreach organization devoted to promoting the health of the Ethiopian immigrants in Israel—the only organization in Israel dedicated to this goal. It was established in 1999 with the purpose of serving the unique cultural and social needs of the Ethiopian immigrants in Israel. Its mission and activities center on the importance of respecting the Ethiopian immigrants' traditions regarding their culture and health beliefs. It conducts health-promotion workshops, seminars, and events for community members in a variety of community settings and it produces a widely popular (and the only) radio program on health in Amharic for the National Radio Broadcast Authority.

An anecdote that illustrates both the opportunities and challenges of the peace building through health work of HATD

Representatives of each of these above three groups (an Ethiopian Jew, a Palestinian from Israel, and a Palestinian from the OPT) met once at an unusual event held at the Jewish Funder's Network (JFN) annual meeting. As its title implies, the JFN is an association of Jewish funders from around the world. In 2012, for the first time, the JFN held its annual meeting in Israel. I (Norbert Goldfield) was the co-chair of the health care track for the conference. I devoted part of that day to the three initiatives described below. There were several remarkable aspects to the meeting, which took place in Tira, a Palestinian town in Israel. The leader of the Ethiopian organization had lived very close to Tira for more than twenty years, yet this was his first visit to the Palestinian Israeli town of Tira. While all three representatives, on hearing each other's presentations, remarked on the similarity of the social and economic challenges they faced, the additional political and resultant health care challenges that Palestinians living in the OPT faced were not discussed. And, tellingly, the organizers of the JFN meeting were concerned about safety for Jews traveling to a Palestinian town, even one in Israel. Security vehicles accompanied the bus—both in front and in back—carrying JFN members.

Results of the interventions

PMRS

In this quality improvement intervention, type 2 diabetic patients were followed up for six months.[17] Each of these patients was registered at primary care clinics operated by the PMRS in three Occupied Palestinian Territory (OPT) villages. A total number of 287 patients, drawn from the same three villages, were included in the program. Aboud (51 patients) is close to Ramallah, Singil (48 patients) is a bit farther north on the road to Nablus, while Ithna (188 patients) is a considerable distance from Ramallah and is west of Hebron, near the border with Israel. At the time of this initiative (2004–6), travel in and out of these villages was typically very difficult, as the Israeli army had deposited boulders and other debris at principal entry points. Patients who were included in the program received free laboratory testing, were offered medical checkups on a monthly basis, and were targeted by a structured health promotion program addressing key self-management behaviors. Health promotion, implemented by community health workers (CHW) (at that time, the PMRS had its own CHW "training school," which provided three years of formal training), utilized different techniques to support patients in an effort to increase social support. These interventions include:

- organizing support groups for patients, their families, and staff members;
- scheduling regular and more frequent medical office visits/ laboratory tests;
- scheduling regular and more frequent staff visits to patient homes.

Laboratory results on these almost 300 participants demonstrated a decrease in the HgbA1c, or Hemoglobin A1c (this number, which measures the average amount of sugar in the blood, indicates diabetes control over a month; a lower number is better), from 9.2 to 8.5 (that is, from "poor" to "good," but not to "excellent"). Participants in Singil realized the greatest improvement, with almost 90% of them showing a lower HgbA1c after the intervention.

The Galilee Society

This initiative was conducted in an Arab-Muslim town in Northern Israel to assess the level of knowledge, beliefs, concerns about diabetes care, and to what extent the care is affected by financial constraints. A questionnaire was administered, and more than a third of respondents reported not receiving any counseling on issues such as foot care or the effects of smoking on diabetes; misconceptions attributable to social norms were common; and more than a third went without taking medications for financial reasons. The results also revealed that respondents had inaccurate knowledge or misconceptions regarding diabetes, including medication use and the effects of diet on the condition. The majority of respondents (56%) believed (incorrectly) that honey consumption does not affect blood glucose levels and that diabetes is a disease of persons who are financially well off (85%). Only 25% of respondents answered correctly 5 or more of the 8 questions pertaining to diabetes.[18]

These results were gathered at the end of the first year of the intervention and presented at a "diabetes study day," attended by staff members of the Galilee Society, myself, and health professionals from other constituency groups, such as Kupat Holim Clalit, a local managed care organization (MCO). At the conclusion of the study day, I made the following recommendations to the senior Galilee Society leadership:

- ask the MCO to support a project that would eliminate or drastically reduce copayments for diabetic patients and document how that might impact health;
- ask the MCO to help fund a community educator who could work with a group of diabetics as described under the next bullet;
- organize a group of diabetics who are knowledgeable/have reasonable control of their diabetes. This group of well-controlled diabetics in turn could work with a much larger group of diabetics in Tamra to help the latter group with diabetes control, exercise, or any of the items identified as barriers to diabetes control in Tamra. Put differently, I suggested that part of the role of the Galilee Society should be to educate a group of leaders who are diabetic. I could see some of these "empowered" diabetics become so excited about civic involvement that they would get involved in the Galilee Society.

The program with the Galilee Society did not continue after the first year of funding. As discussed below, Healing Across the Divides confronted two challenges: most important, we had unrealistic expectations as to how long it would take to form working relations with the established health care system (for example, the local MCOs). Second, and similar to the challenge confronted by Tene Briut (see below), the Galilee Society had difficulty moving from an individual one-on-one interaction with diabetics participating in the program to a group approach. The individual approach became prohibitively expensive, as engaging with individuals was expensive in and of itself, and lack of coordination with the already existing Israeli health care system made some of the services duplicative. The fact that the *kupot* are not used to working with (and in some ways preferred not to work with) NGOs such as the Galilee Society only exacerbated these challenges.

Tene Briut

Tene Briut tried to implement a program very similar to that of both the Galilee Society and the PMRS. That is, Tene Briut, in cooperation with the major MCO serving the Ethiopians, identified a neighborhood with a large number of older, chronically unstable diabetic Ethiopian patients. A specially trained Tene Briut health instructor was to visit patients at home, establish a personal connection, identify individual obstacles to medication compliance, deliver core health information pertaining to diabetes, and involve the family in supporting the diabetic patient. There were also to be weekly group meetings to provide information on medication, disease management, and the vital importance of good nutrition and regular physical activity. In addition, patients were to be encouraged to walk together for exercise on a regular basis with Tene Briut volunteers.

While fine in theory, the Tene Briut program in practice suffered from the same challenges as the Galilee Society initiative. Chief among them, HATD was still too young an organization to appreciate the complexities of getting a community-based initiative off the ground, especially in a First World country like Israel. That is, unlike the PMRS, operating in a Third World country under military occupation, which could deliver care until recently without significant governmental interference, both the Galilee Society and Tene Briut had to operate within the boundaries of an already existing health care system. To put it simply, the established health care system was not interested in working with community-based organizations. The MCOs felt they were already doing a fine job, patient confidentiality had to be respected, and turf issues abounded. Even more important, we realized that we did not have a systematic scientifically validated approach to community engagement with diabetics. Or, as Kate Lorig, the developer of the Stanford Chronic Disease Self-Management Program (CDSMP), has observed:

> It is important to distinguish between "Evidence-Based" as defined above and "based on evidence." Most health education programs are based on evidence [such as the ones of Tene Briut and the Galilee Society: author's note]. That is, the content they teach is factually correct. However, this does not mean that the programs are effective in changing health behaviors. Furthermore, even if effective, a program may not qualify as being evidence based. For example, a diabetes program may reduce A1C under controlled conditions, but may be impractical or impossible to implement on a widespread basis. Barriers may include cost, lack of qualified personnel, lack of fidelity, or unacceptability to a large percentage of the population.[19]

The Stanford Chronic Disease Self-Management Program provided the scientific and effective approach that HATD was looking for.

The Chronic Disease Self-Management Program (CDSMP)

In working to improve the health of diabetics or anyone with a chronic lifelong illness (obesity, headaches, arthritis, heart failure, depression), health professionals must consider the following questions:

- Who is best able to communicate needed activities of daily living, including diet, nutrition, exercise?
- Who is best able to work with individuals for improvement in the control of the chronic illness?

The answer is not just one person. There needs to be a team approach. That team needs to include lay people, preferably people who have a chronic illness, such as diabetes. Such an intervention can result in improved self-management, confidence, and empowerment.

Self-management relates to the tasks that an individual must undertake to live well with one or more chronic conditions. Primary among these tasks is gaining confidence to deal with medical management, role management, and emotional management. It should be noted that self-management refers to both skills and confidence. The skills called for can vary, depending on the condition. Confidence is defined as empowerment or as self-efficacy, the belief that one can accomplish a specific behavior.[20]

The CDSMP is best described by its developer, Professor Kate Lorig:

> The Chronic Disease Self-Management Program, CDSMP, is a six-week community-based workshop to assist people living with one or more chronic condition to improve their skills in medical, role, and emotional management. It is usually taught by peer leaders who receive 24 hours of standardized training. Subjects covered include:
>
> - Techniques to deal with problems such as frustration, fatigue, pain, and isolation.
> - Appropriate exercise for maintaining and improving strength, flexibility, and endurance.

- Appropriate use of medications.
- Communicating effectively with family, friends, and health professionals.
- Managing depression.
- Better breathing techniques.
- Relaxation techniques.
- Healthy eating habits.
- Making good decisions about your health.
- How to evaluate new treatments.[21]

The CDSMP directly addresses the issues of cost, lack of qualified personnel, native-language accessibility, and lack of fidelity that we confronted in our first initiatives with the PMRS, the Galilee Society, and Tene Briut. Significant research literature has demonstrated the reliability and validity of the CDSMP. For example, in 2019 a randomized trial of a weight-loss intervention to prevent diabetes among low-income Hispanics proved effective:

> We recruited overweight/obese adults from more than 50 community sites and conducted oral glucose tolerance testing and completed other clinical assessments and a health and lifestyle survey. We randomized pre-diabetic participants to intervention or delayed intervention groups. Intervention participants attended eight 90-minute peer-led workshop sessions at community sites. Participants in both groups returned for follow-up assessments 6 months after randomization. The main outcomes were the proportion of participants who achieved 5% weight loss, percentage weight loss, and change in the probability of developing diabetes over the next 7.5 years according to the San Antonio Diabetes Prediction Model. We enrolled 402 participants who were mainly female (85%), Latino (73%) or Black (23%), foreign-born (64%), and non-English-speaking (58%). At 6 months, the intervention group had lost a greater percentage of their baseline weight, had a significantly lower rise in HbA1c (glycated hemoglobin), decreased risk of diabetes, larger decreases in fat and fiber intake, improved confidence in nutrition label reading, and decrease in sedentary behavior as compared with the control group. Thus, in partnership with community stakeholders, we created an

effective low-resource program that was less intensive than previously studied programs by incorporating strategies to engage and affect our priority population.[22]

The editor of this book and one of its co-authors, Norbert Goldfield, became a master trainer in the program and has personally trained the trainers from ABBC, Caritas, Diabetes Palestine, and the FDS.

The last three CDSMP-focused interventions: the implementing institutions

Caritas Jerusalem, founded in 1967 in the aftermath of the Six-Day War, is a humanitarian and development organization that represents the socio-pastoral services of the Catholic Church in the Occupied Palestinian Territory. Its mission is to enhance the quality and accessibility of social and medical services for the poor and marginalized; ensure food security; create economic opportunities through soft loan schemes and job creation; provide emergency humanitarian aid on a daily basis; empower youth as community leaders; and advocate for peace, freedom, and justice in the Holy Land. Caritas Jerusalem operates in East Jerusalem, the West Bank, and the Gaza Strip. Its Health Department runs three health centers: two in the West Bank villages of Taybeh and Aboud and one in Gaza.

Ahli Balatah Al-Balad Club (ABBC) was established in Nablus in 1995 by a group of youths to serve young people who were deprived of many basic services at that time. ABBC's mission is to provide sports and social and cultural services to women, young people, and children in Nablus governorate, especially those in underserved communities. The club offers social, cultural, and psychological support to citizens through its network with other official and non-official bodies in Nablus. It focuses on education, health, and psychosocial support as strategic development fields for improving the living conditions in the area.

Diabetes Palestine (DP) is a not-for-profit association established in 2005 in the OPT. It operates in both the West Bank and Gaza Strip. DP provides essential services in partnership with main health care providers in Palestine, including the Palestinian Ministry of Health (MoH), the United Nations Relief and Works Agency (UNRWA), and NGOs. DP became a full member of the IDF (International Diabetes Federation) in 2015 and was recognized by the IDF as a center of excellence.

Results of the last three interventions using the CDSMP

The program with Diabetes Palestine—the first initiative we are funding in Gaza, which we are very excited about—is at its beginning stages, with no results yet to report.

ABBC has just completed its second year, and the preliminary results, after working with several hundred participants, are as follows:

- 12% of the beneficiaries displayed reduced blood sugars.
- 81% of the beneficiaries gave clear statements about positive improvement in their psychological health.
- 81% of the beneficiaries reported a positive change in their eating habits.
- 69% of the beneficiaries got no physical exercise before the project and perform at least one physical exercise per week as a result of the sessions.
- 73% of the beneficiaries report increased social activities with their families and society as a whole.

Just as important, as discussed below, ABBC has established a working relationship with the Palestinian Ministry of Health (MoH).

The key activities for Caritas were:

- November 2017: Training Caritas Staff in Stanford Chronic Disease Self-Management Program (CDSMP).
- Caritas staff trained 15 village health activators in CDSMP.
- Screening people who are older than 35 years in the following villages: Aboud, Karawa, Kuforain, Der Abu Meshal, Al-Nabi Salah, Nallin, Shuqba, Bat Reema, Dar Ghassanih, and Qibia. In this process, individuals with chronic diseases who would like to participate in the Stanford CDSMP were identified.
- 15 village health activators trained 375 individuals with chronic diseases in Stanford CDSMP.

- Following up lab tests on hypertensive and diabetic patients and conducting lab tests.
- Observing change in resilience of participating individuals utilizing the Stanford CDSMP and home visits (more than 6,000 home visits).
- Evaluating the program through pre- and post-intervention questionnaires using the Dartmouth COOP charts.

Three hundred and seventy-five individuals completed the pre- and post-intervention questionnaires in the Caritas initiative. While only one item, quality of life, is shown in Figure 3.1, the results were similar for all 9 items: they conveyed an important improvement

Q 5: Quality of life

			Order of the Questionnaires			Total
			Pre-test	After 6 months	After 12 months	
Quality of life	Very well; could hardly be better	Count	5	19	51	75
		% Within Quality of life	4.6%	13.8%	81.6%	100.0%
	Pretty good	Count	60	185	161	406
		% Within Quality of life	11.0%	32.7%	56.2%	100.0%
	Good and bad parts about equal	Count	318	402	248	968
		% Within Quality of life	33.3%	41.4%	25.3%	100.0%
	Pretty bad	Count	170	88	23	281
		% Within Quality of life	61.4%	30.3%	8.3%	100.0%
	Very bad; could hardly be worse	Count	140	13	7	160
		% Within Quality of life	91.3%	5.8%	2.9%	100.0%

Figure 3.1 Change in quality of life over time (12 months)

(although not tested for statistical significance) in not just quality of life but also lower pain, better overall health, improved social support, and reduced depression.

Overall summary, lessons learned, and future possibilities

Measurable health improvement is possible with any of the interventions described in this chapter. It is very likely that long-lasting individual change can occasionally occur with any evidence-based method. However, long-lasting change both at the individual level for large groups of people and at the organizational level is possible only with programs such as the CDSMP. While there are other evidence-based interventions that can impact large groups of people, only the CDSMP has been translated and validated in Arabic. Thus, when I do a training of trainers using the CDSMP, the new trainers have a manual at their disposal in their native language that they can use when they train 25 diabetics in CDSMP.

Using the CDSMP, organizational capacity building has occurred in several ways. It has provided a "language" of communication between organizations. For example, the Family Defense Society (FDS; see Chapter 7), Caritas, and ABBC have exchanged ideas and worked together on the basis that they were utilizing similar programmatic interventions (although each organization supplemented the CDSMP with its own material and added significant changes to the programmatic intervention). ABBC, based in Nablus, has begun to exchange information with the Diabetes Palestine intervention located in Gaza. HATD staff on the ground will foster this interaction but, in line with our organizational philosophy, we will not insist on it.

Sustainability of interventions in the OPT is very challenging for many reasons, as discussed in other chapters; economic, logistical, political, and other factors come into play. In light of these challenges, I am particularly pleased that ABBC, in particular, and also FDS have established a working relationship with the Palestinian Ministry of Health (MoH). How far that will go is unclear at the present time. An ideal, for example, would be for ABBC and FDS leadership to work with the MoH and train 30 new CDSMP trainers, including several MoH leaders.

The work carried out with Caritas and Diabetes Palestine brings up the question: Are they community-based organizations? Caritas decidedly is not. Diabetes Palestine, the equivalent of the American Diabetes Association in the United States, was located on the grounds of the Augusta Victoria Hospital, the largest referral center for Palestinians in the OPT. The HATD board discusses on an ongoing basis the line between "true" community-based organizations and organizations such as Caritas and Diabetes Palestine (DP). ABBC is a local sports club; Caritas is part of the Catholic Church. DP is affiliated with the International Diabetes Federation. While Caritas and DP are not true community-based organizations, we had hoped that Caritas, for example, would, after a successful intervention, not only be interested in working with the Palestinian MoH but also seek funds from other Caritas groups throughout the world and form relationships with them. For reasons that are not clear to me, Caritas did not pursue this option, including trying to work with Caritas groups in other countries, for support and sharing of the excellent work that they did. HATD stopped funding the intervention after two years despite the fact that the work that the organization did was exemplary.

Concluding comments: an anecdote and a comment on the relationship between self-management, self-confidence, and political empowerment

While on the surface the first two Israeli initiatives undertaken by Healing Across the Divides seemed unsuccessful, the engagement between the two organizations that occurred after the completion of their initiatives validated the work we did together. Tene Briut decided to join a lawsuit that the Galilee Society filed against the Israeli government alleging discrimination on the basis of race and income. The joint meetings that HATD had facilitated between all HATD grantees, including the Galilee Society, led to Tene Briut's decision. I (Norbert Goldfield) happened to attend the Tene Briut meeting in which they decided to join the lawsuit. The anecdote that I most recall from this conversation was the unanimous sentiment from the Tene Briut staff that Ethiopian Jews were discriminated against by other Israelis in a way not too dissimilar from the treatment of Palestinians in Israel, and thus Tene Briut should join the lawsuit. They won the lawsuit.

In an effort to impact the ever-widening scourge of diabetes in Israel and the OPT, Healing across the Divides has funded numerous initiatives addressing this chronic illness. Our impact was initially limited largely through lack of fidelity to validated interventions. Using the CDSMP addressed all the challenges that we faced in our first interventions. In this situation, "fidelity" refers not only to a standardized curriculum in combination with the mode of delivery but also the critical fact that the entire course has been translated and validated in Arabic, and it is anticipated that the CDSMP will be translated into Hebrew in 2021. The course clearly has resulted in improved self-management and self-confidence for hundreds of diabetics.

But what about empowerment? There are two aspects of this term. "Empowerment" can describe the confidence of a diabetic teen living in Gaza to say to his parents that he needs to be able to decide what food he or she wishes to eat. The question, I ask myself, is whether or not there is any way for a community-based group implementing this self-management program to incorporate other messages that will result in the diabetic teen asserting that he or she has the right to adequate medication and supplies for the effective treatment of his or her illness. Put differently, Kate Lorig, the developer of the CDSMP, in turn quoted Dr. Tom Ferguson, who said that "doctors (health professionals) would get off their pedestals when patients got off their knees."[23] All of us, patients, health professionals, community-based organizations, and health care organizations, should do a bit more to adjust our political "posture." That is, we all must consider to what extent the term "empowerment" in community-based health interventions can be broadened to include health and, even, political rights. Diabetic teens and health professionals in Israel and the OPT need to be empowered in every sense of the term, and Healing Across the Divides continues to explore ways that we can achieve that through community-based interventions. These are some of the political (in its broad application) implications of the diabetes interventions that HATD has sponsored and funded.

Notes

1   Please see https://www.selfmanagementresource.com/programs/small-group/
    chronic-disease-self-management for more information. Accessed: June 3, 2020.
2   Joslin, EP. (1921) The prevention of diabetes mellitus. *JAMA*, 76 (2), p. 79.
    Available at: https://jamanetwork.com/journals/jama/article-abstract/226259.
    Accessed: June 3, 2020.
3   Kaiser, AB., Zhang, N., Van Der Puum, W., (2018) Global Prevalence of Type
    2 Diabetes over the Next Ten Years - 2018-2028 *Diabetes 67* (Supplement 1)
    Available at: https://diabetes.diabetesjournals.org/content/67/Supplement_1/
    202-LB. Accessed: June 3, 2020.
4   Dewa, C., Cimo, A. (2018). Symptoms of mental illness and their impact
    on managing type 2 diabetes in adults. *Can J Diabetes* 42(4), pp: 372–381.
    Available at: https://pubmed.ncbi.nlm.nih.gov/29128304/?from_term=mental+
    health+and+diabetes&from_page=2&from_pos=3. Accessed: June 3, 2020.
5   Picard, M., McEwan, B. (2018) Psychological stress and mitochondria: a con-
    ceptual framework. *Psychosom Med.* 80(2): pp: 126–140. Available at: https://
    www.ncbi.nlm.nih.gov/pmc/articles/PMC5901651/. Accessed: June 3, 2020.
6   Jaffe, A., Giveon, S., Wulffhart, L., Oberman, B., Baidousi M., et al.
    (2017) Adult Arabs have higher risk for diabetes mellitus than Jews in Israel.
    PLOS ONE 12(5): e0176661. Available at: https://doi.org/10.1371/journal.
    pone.0176661. Accessed: June 3, 2020.
7   Na'amnih, W., Muhsen, K., Tarabeia, J., et al. (2010). Trends in the gap in life
    expectancy between Arabs and Jews in Israel between 1975 and 2004. *Interna-
    tional Journal of Epidemiology.* 39 (5) pp: 1324–1332. Available at: https://www.
    researchgate.net/publication/44660262_ Accessed: June 3, 2020.
8   Baron-Epel, O., Garty, N., & Green, M. S. (2007). Inequalities in use of
    health services among Jews and Arabs in Israel. *Health Services Research*, *42*
    (3 Pt 1), pp: 1008–1019. Available at: https://www.ncbi.nlm.nih.gov/pmc/articles/
    PMC1955256/. Accessed: June 3, 2020.
9   Baron-Epel, O., Keinan-Boker, L., Weinstein, R., et al. (2010) Persistent high
    rates of smoking among Israeli Arab males with concomitant decrease among
    Jews. *Isr Med Assoc J.* 2010;12(12) pp: 732–737. Available at: https://pubmed.
    ncbi.nlm.nih.gov/21348400/. Accessed: June 3, 2020.
10 Abu-Rmeileh, NM., Husseini, A., O'Flaherty, M., Shoaibi, A., Capewell, S.
    (2012) Forecasting prevalence of type 2 diabetes mellitus in Palestinians to
    2030: validation of a predictive model. *Lancet* 380:S21. Available at: https://
    www.thelancet.com/journals/lancet/article/PIIS0140-6736(13)60202-0/
    fulltext. Accessed: June 3, 2020.
11 Abu Al-Halaweh, A., Almdal, T., O'Rourke, N., et al. (2019). Mobile care
    teams improve metabolic control for adults with Type II diabetes in the South-
    ern West Bank, Palestine. *Diabetes and Metabolic Syndrome Clinical Research
    and Reviews.* 13, pp: 782–785. Available at: https://www.researchgate.net/
    publication/329353316_Mobile_care_teams_improve_metabolic_control_
    for_adults_with_Type_II_diabetes_in_the_Southern_West_Bank_Palestine.
    Accessed: June 3, 2020.
12 Velo, P. (2016) Killing them slowly: diabetes in Palestine life under Israeli
    occupation has spurred the progress of diabetes, the leading indirect cause of
    death in Palestine. *Al Jazeera News.* https://www.aljazeera.com/news/2016/07/
    killing-slowly-diabetes-palestine-160728085301648.html.Accessed: June 3, 2020.
13 Quoted in http://www.tene-briut.org.il/index.php/en/health-and-the-ethiopian-
    israeli-community. Accessed: June 3, 2020.

14 Quoted in http://www.tene-briut.org.il/index.php/en/health-and-the-ethiopian-israeli-community. Accessed: June 3, 2020.

15 Jaffe, A., Giveon, S., Wulffhart, L., et al. (2016). Diabetes among Ethiopian immigrants to Israel: exploring the effects of migration and ethnicity on diabetes risk. *PLOS ONE, 11*(6), e0157354. Available at: https://journals.plos.org/plosone/article?id=10.1371/journal.pone.0157354. Accessed: June 3, 2020.

16 https://en.wikipedia.org/wiki/2005_Palestinian_presidential_election.

17 Abu Ghosh, H., Shaar, A., Mashal, J., et al. (2007) Diabetes Control in Three Villages: A Community-Based Quality Improvement Intervention. *Journal of Ambulatory Care Management*. 30 (1), pp: 74–78.

18 Khatib, M., Efrat, S., Deeb, D. (2007) Knowledge, beliefs, and economic barriers to healthcare: a survey of diabetic patients in an Arab-Israeli town, *Journal of Ambulatory Care Management*. 30 (1), pp: 79–85.

19 Lorig, K. (2017). Commentary on "Evidence-based self-management programs for seniors and other with chronic diseases": patient experience—patient health—return on investment. *Journal of Ambulatory Care Management*. 40 (3), pp: 185–188.

20 Wasson, J., Coleman, EA. (2014) Health confidence: an essential measure for patient engagement and better practice. *Fam Pract Manag*. 21(5), pp: 8–12.

21 Available at https://www.cdc.gov/learnmorefeelbetter/programs/general.htm. Accessed: June 3, 2020.

22 Lorig, K.R. Sobel, DS., Stewart, A., (1999) Evidence suggesting that a chronic disease self-management program can improve health status while reducing utilization and costs: A randomized trial. *Medical Care*, 37(1), pp: 5–14.

23 Mayer, V.L., Vangeepuram, N., Fei, K., et al. (2019) Outcomes of a weight loss intervention to prevent diabetes among low-income residents of East Harlem, New York. *Health Educ Behav*. 46(6), pp: 1073–1082. Available at: https://www.ncbi.nlm.nih.gov/pmc/articles/PMC6908807/pdf/nihms-1061994.pdf. Accessed: June 3, 2020.

Chapter 4

Al-Maqdese

Drug abuse prevention among Palestinian youth in East Jerusalem

Isam Jwihan, Gada Muhsin, Nael Hasan,
Norbert Goldfield and Richard A. Rawson

Introduction

In November 2017, the Palestine National Institute of Public Health (PNIMH) completed a study to determine the prevalence of illicit drug use in the Occupied Palestinian Territory (OPT).[1] The study estimated that there were 26,500 high-risk drug users (HRDU) in the OPT, which constituted 1.8% of the male population aged 15 and above. Hashish/marijuana and synthetic marijuana were the drugs used most in the West Bank, whereas the prescription drugs tramadol and Lyrica (pregabalin) were the most used in Gaza. The percentage of HRDU who ever injected drugs in the West Bank is much higher than that in Gaza, 8% versus 2%, respectively. A major recommendation of the PNIMH study was the implementation of a drug abuse prevention program. This chapter summarizes the three-year implementation of Unplugged, an evidence-based drug abuse prevention program, with Palestinian high school students in East Jerusalem. In the introduction, we describe the Unplugged program and provide background on the organization implementing the initiative and brief geopolitical background to the geographic area where the initiative was implemented. This chapter then consists of methods, followed by results, and concludes with a discussion.

Unplugged is a school-based curriculum following a social-influence model that aims to decrease drug use among high school students. The program involves students, school staff, and parents. In a randomized trial conducted in Europe, implementation of Unplugged was associated with "lower prevalence of daily use of cigarettes, episodes of drunkenness, and cannabis use in the [previous] 30 days."[2] Researchers have translated the Unplugged program into Arabic.[3]

This chapter reports on an innovative training program for Unplugged and the subsequent delivery of the Unplugged program to Palestinian high school youth living in East Jerusalem. Al-Maqdese for Society Development (hereafter referred to as Al-Maqdese), a local Palestinian community organization, implemented Unplugged in this project and is continuing to implement the program.[4] A civic nonprofit and non-governmental organization (NGO) established in Jerusalem on February 19, 2007, Al-Maqdese has as its mission to protect and defend Palestinians' rights, ensure respect for the rule of law, and promote the principles of democracy in the Occupied Palestinian Territory (OPT).

It is important to consider the background of this program implementation in East Jerusalem. The Israeli-Palestinian conflict is one of the oldest ongoing conflicts in the world today. After the British left what was then Palestine, the Jordanians controlled East Jerusalem from 1948 to 1967. Since the June War of 1967, Israel has controlled East Jerusalem and has formally annexed it without international recognition, except for that of the United States. The Palestinian National Authority (PNA), established in 1994 after the Oslo Accords between Israel and the Palestinians, has nominal control over parts of the West Bank but not East Jerusalem. Nonetheless, the PNA Ministry of Education, based in Ramallah, plays an informal role in the education of Palestinian youth in East Jerusalem. Al-Maqdese, at the present time, looks to the PNA for guidance on educational matters. Conversely, Al-Maqdese has an impact on the PNA Ministry of Education, setting the stage for possible implementation of Unplugged at least throughout the West Bank.

Initially, Al-Maqdese proposed to implement the DARE program.[5] However, in view of the absence of empirical support for DARE and after consultation with the funding organization and an international expert, Al-Maqdese staff very willingly implemented the Unplugged program instead.

Implementing social interventions of any kind in a setting of ongoing conflict faces enormous hurdles. During the period of implementation of this initiative, many houses inhabited by Palestinians in East Jerusalem were demolished by the Israeli government,[6, 7, 8] there were (and still are) ongoing efforts by Israeli nationalists to take over homes inhabited by Palestinians in East Jerusalem,[9] and numerous clashes occurred frequently between Israeli Jews and Palestinians. These events created problems with the implementation of the Unplugged program. In addition, Al-Maqdese experienced relatively frequent personnel changes. Despite these challenges, Al-Maqdese successfully implemented the Unplugged program.

This chapter describes how a distance-learning method using Skype and an Arabic-speaking trainer effectively provided a training program to give the Palestinian team the knowledge and skills to deliver Unplugged. Following the training, the trainers delivered the Unplugged program as designed to students, teachers, and family members. This chapter also discusses the impact of the Unplugged program on these individuals.

Methods

Implementation

Senior staff at the Al-Maqdese organization in Jerusalem recognized the need to address increasing drug use among Palestinian youth. In response, they submitted an application to Healing Across the Divides (HATD) to provide a prevention program based on the DARE (Drug Abuse Resistance Education) program used in some parts of the United States. After discussions between HATD and Al-Maqdese, it was decided to fund Al-Maqdese to conduct a prevention program using the Unplugged curriculum as the evidence-based program. This process took approximately one year and involved site visits and a review of Al-Maqdese's published material. As part of the agreement to fund the initiative, HATD arranged for an introductory lecture on evidence-based approaches to substance-abuse prevention by Richard A. Rawson, professor at the UCLA Geffen School of Medicine. As the training for Unplugged had to be done in Arabic, it was necessary to find an Arabic-speaking professional trained in Unplugged. Dr. Nael Hasan, an Egyptian psychiatrist living in Abu Dhabi who specializes in substance abuse treatment, is one of the few Arabic-speaking professionals trained in Unplugged. Dr. Hasan was part of the team in Abu Dhabi that translated the Unplugged curriculum into Arabic. Initially, an in-person training program for Palestinian trainers was considered; however, because travel by Arab professionals to East

Jerusalem is difficult, if not impossible, with barriers presently placed by Israeli and Abu Dhabi travel restrictions, HATD and Al-Maqdese, together with Dr. Hasan, elected to try to conduct the Unplugged training via Skype, an app that enables video connections between computers and other information technology platforms.

On completion of the training (described below), Al-Maqdese implemented the program in twelve high schools in East Jerusalem. Their selection was based on several factors, including the absence of such programs at the time and the schools' location in an area lacking Israeli or Palestinian police and thus classified as dangerous, with an attendant high rate of crime, particularly, the proximity of drugs and drug dealers to the schools. These schools, in areas outside the wall surrounding Jerusalem, are isolated, neglected, underserviced, and have a large student population. The Palestinian Directorate of Education recognized these schools as more in need of the Unplugged type of program than those in other areas. Finally, Al-Maqdese wanted to focus on schools where it was already conducting other support projects.

In accordance with the Unplugged program, in addition to high school students who went through the Unplugged sessions, parents, school counselors, and teachers also participated. Moreover, in an effort to promote sustainability, Al-Maqdese also involved personnel from the Ministries of Education and Police.

Design

HATD, together with Al-Maqdese and Dr. Hasan, arranged for the Skype training. It consisted of six Skype sessions and two booster/fidelity sessions. Each of the six sessions, approximately 45 to 60 minutes long, reviewed two of the Unplugged weekly topics/ exercises. The Palestinian representative of Healing Across the Divides attended all of the Skype training sessions. Although participants were involved in and completed all the sessions, the Internet connection proved somewhat unreliable, which led to many interruptions. After every session, Al-Maqdese staff sent a report by email to all the participants and anyone who could not attend the sessions. Attendance was taken to document trainer participation.

Al-Maqdese staff who had completed the training began to implement the Unplugged program in fall 2016, at the beginning of the academic year, among the students. Separately, they trained parents and counselors to be effective change agents of drug abuse prevention with their teenage children and/or students, as recommended in the Unplugged program. Representatives of Healing Across the Divides and the PNA Ministries of Education and Police observed some of the sessions in the school (PNA Ministry of Education) or had informal conversations about the trainings with other groups, such as parents, who participated in the program.

The Unplugged program consists of twelve 60-minute sessions with students in their schools. The 1,200 participating students, all Muslim and of both sexes, ranged in age from 14 to 16 and were equally divided between grades 8, 9, and 10.

The participation of parents, mentors, and teachers was complementary to the student sessions. The training of parents aimed at influencing children's behavior by changing parents' beliefs, raising their awareness, and promoting dialogue and discussion, as well as educating them on positive parenting techniques and strategies. The parents attended three meetings, each of which lasted more than two hours. Among the topics related to their adolescent children discussed during these meetings were how to understand adolescents better and clarifying societal "rules" and laws that regulate the relationship of parents and their children. The training of mentors and teachers focused on how to use the program materials effectively with students. These meetings benefited from more modern training techniques than were used in other sessions, such as films and pictures, group distribution, reality simulation, role-playing, brainstorming, and interactive discussion. As it was interactive, the training of teachers required a longer period than that of parents.

Data

In the three years of the Unplugged program, more than a thousand students in twelve schools (eight high schools and four middle schools) participated in the Unplugged program. In addition, 70 teachers and counselors and 100 parents participated in separate programs.

Two different questionnaires were fielded. The first was an Arabic translation (by Mentor Arabia) of the questionnaire that was developed for the initial European trials of Unplugged.[10] A pre- and post-intervention questionnaire completed by 125 students was collected and analyzed. When input from the Al-Maqdese trainers and students indicated that the questionnaire was too long and asked many unimportant or culturally irrelevant questions, a shorter version was developed by Al-Maqdese staff, together with United States and Egyptian experts. In year 3, 75 students completed this shorter questionnaire before and after their participation in Unplugged. This study reports on data from that 75-student sample. The shorter questionnaire used a number of the questions from the original questionnaire with exactly the same wording. These original items are analyzed in the following "Results" section. The English and Arabic versions of the questionnaire are available on request.

In addition to the questionnaire data, qualitative narratives were collected by Al-Maqdese from students, parents, counselors, the HATD representative, and the Ministries of Education and Police, from not only the schools in East Jerusalem but also the additional trainings that the Palestinian Ministries of Education and Police asked Al-Maqdese to conduct in other locations in the West Bank, such as Hebron. HATD staff attended several of the Al-Maqdese sessions with students and parents.

Data management and analysis

Al-Maqdese collected the quantitative information contained in the questionnaires and entered the data into Excel spreadsheets. Al-Maqdese staff prepared a preliminary analysis of the data. This was complemented by analyses conducted by HATD staff.

Outcomes tracked

Three different types of outcomes were tracked in this initiative. Quantitatively, we compared answers to the same pre- and post-intervention questionnaires from the 75-person student sample. Al-Maqdese staff, teachers, and counselors collected qualitative information, including reports of behavior change and case examples with specific students. The extent to which the Ministry of Education adopted the Unplugged program going forward was the third outcome examined.

Results

Sample

In the three years of the Unplugged program, more than a thousand students in twelve schools (eight high school and four middle schools) participated in the Unplugged program. In addition, 70 teachers and counselors and 100 parents participated in separate programs.

Quantitative results

Of 75 respondents to the survey in year 3 of the initiative, 53 were male and 22 female. They largely lived with two parents at home, sharing their bedroom with other siblings. According to question-naire results, smoking was the greatest substance-abuse risk factor.

Drug use questions

A series of questions gave insight into the respondent's opinions of substance abuse. Question 14 queried behavioral intentions to use/not use drugs in the future. Question 17 queried the perceived risk of drug use.

QUESTION 14: When asked, "How likely is it that you will be doing each of the following A YEAR FROM NOW?" (Q14), The pre- and post-Unplugged program responses were contrasted to measure a self-reported change in behavioral intentions. The four possible responses (likelihood) to Q14 were compared across the five sub-stance categories, which were cigarettes, alcoholic beverages, getting drunk, smoking marijuana, taking other illegal substances.

Respondents who reported a change toward less likely use in four of the five categories were identified as being positively impacted by the education program; 20 of the 75 (26.7%) respondents (12 male, 8 female) reported that they were less likely to use substances one year from the time of survey than at the outset of the program. A 99% confidence interval for the rate of impact falls between 14.7% and 41.7%, signifying a significant change. The difference in change rate between males (22.6%) and females (36.4%) was not found to be significant ($P > .05$) at the 95% confidence level.

QUESTION 17: When asked, "How much do you think PEOPLE RISK harming themselves (physically or in other ways)?" (Q17), the pre- and post-Unplugged responses were compared as a measure of change in perceived risk. The four responses to Q17 (no risk, slight risk, great risk, don't know) were consolidated into three categories, with "unknown" set equal to no risk. Post-Unplugged perceived-risk scores were higher than the scores in the pre-test in four of the six drug categories (e.g., smoke cigarettes occasionally, smoke one or more packs of cigarettes a day), suggesting a positive impact by the Unplugged program in the perceived risks of substance use. For Q17, 12 of the 75 (16.0%) respondents (9 male, 3 female) reported that they perceived use of substances as more risky at post-test than at the out-set of the program. A 99% confidence interval for the rate of impact falls between 6.9% and 29.6%, indicating a significant change. The difference in change rate between males (17.0%) and females (13.6%) was not found to be significant (P > .05).

Attendance was taken at the training sessions (the mean number of trainers per session was approximately 25); all of the Al-Maqdese trainers who ultimately delivered the training in schools attended all eight Skype sessions. Further, the entire staff of Al-Maqdese attended the vast majority of the training sessions.

Qualitative results: Case examples

Following are three summaries of accounts collected by Al-Maqdese trainers from staff and students who participated in the Unplugged program.

a   Palestinian students were illegally buying cigarettes from a shop in East Jerusalem. Two students encouraged the rest of the class to smoke by promoting false information about the benefits of smoking. After a number of Unplugged meetings, students were asked to participate in a contest to see who was able to quit smoking. Some managed to stop smoking, with the help of the educational counselor.

b   After participating in the Unplugged program, one ninth-grade student asked the school social worker for assistance in obtaining treatment for his father's drug and alcohol addiction.

c   A student prone to violent behavior also encouraged fellow stu-
    dents to smoke cigarettes and nargila (smoking using a pipe) and
    urged them to not participate in the Unplugged program. His
    father and uncles were then active drug users, and he lived in his
    grandfather's house. This information came to the attention of
    school officials as a consequence of the Unplugged program. The
    school arranged for one-on-one individual counseling with the
    student, and the father and uncles stopped being active drug users
    and some became less violent.

Future implementation results

Al-Maqdese and HATD leaders hoped that the Unplugged project
would generate interest and support for additional implementation
of the Unplugged program beyond the end of the project. Although
this is a continuing effort, to date, it appears that the Ministry of
Education is interested and has supported the following activities
subsequent to the completion of the project.

As of 2019, the following institutions have asked Al-Maqdese for
Unplugged training:

a   The Shofat Palestinian refugee camp: 50 teachers;
b   Al Quds University: 31 teachers through the Community Action
    Center;
c   Modern University College, Ramallah: Social Service Department;
d   The Ministry of Education: contract with Al-Maqdese to train
    30 teachers in 20 schools in Hebron. In addition, separately,
    30 Palestinian police officers from both Ramallah and Hebron
    received lectures on the Unplugged program.

Discussion

Drug abuse is a significant and increasing problem among Palestinian
youth. Interventions using evidence-based programs need to be innovative in light of the continuing Israeli-Palestinian conflict. This
chapter provides preliminary data on the impact of an evidence-based
drug abuse prevention intervention among Palestinian high school

students in East Jerusalem in which those implementing the program were trained through Skype. Current data results document the positive impact of the intervention on the likelihood of these youth smoking (the most common drug use) one year from now.

Al-Maqdese staff were trained in Unplugged, an evidence-based approach, using Skype, an innovative method, in an effort to counteract travel restrictions for Palestinians. In turn, Al-Maqdese staff worked over three years in twelve schools with over a thousand students, approximately 100 parents, and 70 teachers and counselors. In addition, Al-Maqdese conducted training-the-trainer programs with 30 parents of students participating in Unplugged, 25 teachers and social workers, and 30 students. Al-Maqdese has created a marketing plan for the Unplugged program in an effort to disseminate the program throughout the Occupied Palestinian Territory. Finally, attesting to the acceptance of Unplugged, Palestinian authorities in the Ministries of Education and Police have implemented Unplugged in a variety of educational institutions in Ramallah and Hebron. However, funding challenges for these inexpensive initiatives are ongoing. In addition, the political and daily life challenges confronting Palestinians in East Jerusalem continue and, if anything, are worsening.[11]

Acknowledgments

Richard Fuller, MA, conducted the quantitative statistical analysis; Moaz Zateri, general manager of Al-Maqdese, facilitated this initiative.

Notes

1 Palestinian National Institute of Public Health. Estimating the extent of illicit drug use in Palestine. United Nations Office on Drugs and Crime, (2017) *Korea International Cooperation Agency, and World Health Organization*; (internet). Available at: http://www.unodc.org/documents/middleeastandnorthafrica/Publications/Estimating_the_Extent_of_Illicit_Drug_Use_in_Palestine.pdf. Accessed: June 5, 2020.

2 Faggiano, F., Galanti, MR., Bohrn, K. (2008) The effectiveness of a school-based drug abuse prevention program. *PrevMed.* 47 (5) pp: 537–543.

3 European Drug Addiction Prevention Trial. Dissemination area. (2008) *EU-DAP UNODC Romena/Mentor Arabia* (Unplugged translation availability website). Available from: https://www.eudap.net/Dissemination_Unodc_Romena.aspx. Accessed: June 5, 2020

4   Al-Maqdese for Society Development (organization website). Available from: https://www.facebook.com/almaqdese. Accessed: June 5, 2020.

5   West, S. L., & O'Neal, K. K. (2004). Project D.A.R.E. outcome effectiveness revisited. *American Journal of Public Health*, *94*(6), 1027–1029. Available at: https://www.ncbi.nlm.nih.gov/pmc/articles/PMC1448384/pdf/0941027.pdf. Accessed: June 6, 2020.

6   Amnesty International (1999) Israel and the Occupied Territories demolition and dispossession: the destruction of Palestinian homes. https://www.amnesty.org/download/Documents/148000/mde150591999en.pdf.   Accessed: February 7, 2021.

7   Levy, G., Levac, A. (2019) Israel forces Palestinian to raze his and his daughter's homes with his own hands. *Haaretz* Available at: https://www.haaretz.com/israel-news/.premium-israel-forces-palestinian-to-raze-his-and-his-daughter-s-homes-with-his-own-hands-1.7000958. Accessed: June 6, 2020.

8   International Middle East Media Center (2010) Al-Maqdese Concludes Comprehensive Report On Israel's Violations In Jerusalem. Available from: https://imemc.org/article/60044/. Accessed: February 2021.

9   B'Tselem (The Israeli Information Center for Human Rights in the Occupied Territories). East Jerusalem cleansing continues: Israel removes more Palestinian families, hands over their homes to settlers (internet); 2019, March 11. Available from: https://www.btselem.org/jerusalem/20190311_east_jerusalem_cleansing_continues. Accessed: June 6, 2020.

10   personal communication with Dr. Nael Hasan.

11   Sudilovsky, J. (2019) My dream was destroyed': Home demolitions soar in East Jerusalem, P.*972 Magazine* Available at: https://www.972mag.com/east-jerusalem-home-demolitions-settlements/ Accessed: June 6, 2020.

Chapter 5

ASSAF/Israel AIDS Task Force

Promoting equal rights for HIV-positive refugee asylum seekers in Israel

Norbert Goldfield

Introduction

This chapter highlights a conundrum for an organization such as Healing Across the Divides. HATD's mission is to measurably improve the health of marginalized Israelis and Palestinians. What to do about a population that is neither Israeli nor Palestinian? Such a population is not party to nor engaged in the Israeli-Palestinian conflict. Yet members of these populations reside in Israel and are among the most marginalized, if not the most marginalized, people living in this region. For this reason, HATD is engaged with supporting community organizations that, in turn, work to assist the most vulnerable members of the already vulnerable African refugee asylum seekers (RAS) population. Our grants discussed in this chapter have gone to community-based initiatives that focus on those RAS with HIV, many of whom contracted the disease when they were victims of trafficking. This chapter starkly highlights the challenges of humanitarianism, as discussed in chapter 15. It offers introductory comments on the history of the RAS in Israel, followed by summaries of results (and the challenges in obtaining valid data) from four years of interventions with the RAS HIV population. It also summarizes the activities undertaken by the community groups on behalf of the RAS over these four years. The appendix provides a different type of data: six detailed case studies.

African Refugee Asylum Seekers (RAS) in general and in Israel

The 1951 Refugee Convention, of which Israel is a signatory, defines a refugee as someone who "owing to a well-founded fear of being persecuted for reasons of race, religion, nationality, membership of a particular social group or political opinion, is outside the country of his nationality, and is unable to, or owing to such fear, is unwilling to avail himself of the protection of that country."[1] According to the most recent figures, approximately 30,000 asylum seekers live in Israel; of these, 92% are Eritrean and Sudanese.[2] An asylum seeker is a person who has sought protection as a refugee but whose claim for refugee status has not yet been assessed. At its height, there were 70,000 RAS in Israel. Most of these have relocated to either Europe or Canada, with a very small number going to the United States. For a period of time, many RAS men were housed in detention centers (most in one called Holot) in the Negev desert in Southern Israel. As a consequence of a court decision, this was eventually closed down. For a twenty-four-hour period in 2018, the Israeli government negotiated an agreement with the United Nations High Commissioner for Refugees (UNHCR) to give refugee status to 16,000 RAS if the UNHCR would resettle the remainder in third countries.[3] After intense right-wing pushback, the conservative government of Benjamin Netanyahu backtracked and began to take a harder line against the African RAS.

The State of Israel applies today a "nonreturn policy" or "nonde-portation policy," under which the vast majority of asylum seekers from Sudan and Eritrea are granted temporary stay permits that do not confer any rights.[4,5] Through this policy, the government of Israel acknowledges the danger in these countries and does not deport asylum seekers to their countries of origin, especially to countries, such as Sudan and Eritrea, with significant well-documented evidence of widespread systematic torture and other ill treatment. However, the Israeli government continues to offer "voluntary repatriation" to third African countries, such as Rwanda. Very few RAS have accepted the offer.

Without legal status as a refugee, the asylum seekers in Israel are left without rights. Current Israeli policy denies all asylum seekers access to most services. Crucially, the Israeli National Health Insurance Law does not apply to asylum seekers, blocking access to public health services other than in times of medical emergency.

The limbo in which RAS exist leads many to suffer from anxiety, depression, and hopelessness. Their complicated visa status, employment insecurity, lack of social services, and lack of health insurance and access to care are only the tangible challenges asylum seekers experience. Beyond financial and physical pressures, many asylum seekers face a bleak outlook for their personal lives, especially single men whose prospects for achieving stability and establishing families are slim.

HIV and the role of support in well-being for HIV-positive individuals

HIV is a chronic disease whose impact, due to its stigmatized behavior, goes beyond health. A diagnosis of HIV may give rise to difficulties with coping, reduced self-esteem, social isolation, and poorer psychological well-being.[6] Receiving emotional support from significant social network members, such as partners, families, or friends, may mitigate the negative impact of HIV on psychological well-being.[7] Studies have shown that living with HIV generates greater challenges than those posed by many other diseases or conditions, such as levels of depression and stress higher than those for the general population.[8] Higher levels of distress have been associated with riskier health behaviors, including drug use, nonadherence to medication, and unsafe sexual practices,[9] as well as faster disease progression.[10]

Research has found that receiving support from friends, family, and community networks can help to alleviate or prevent psychological distress and promote positive adjustment for people living with HIV.[11] Through empathy and understanding, emotional support provides coping assistance. Greater amounts of emotional support are linked to a more positive affect in people living with HIV.[12] Moreover, people living with HIV who are satisfied with support available to them tend to experience less psychological distress, a higher quality of life, and more self-esteem,[13] while those who perceive low levels of social support experience increased distress.[14]

In the largely "traditional" RAS community, discussing sex and sexually related issues is taboo, which places a high level of stigma on HIV carriers. As many RAS living with HIV or AIDS contracted the disease in the Sinai while being tortured,[15] their illness is associated with the general stigma and shame of being a victim of rape and torture. These individuals are often shunned by and isolated from their friends and community. As a consequence, they often keep their status to themselves, afraid of being judged and ostracized. Moreover, the increased psychological stress caused by this stigma leads many to refrain from reaching out for services that are available to them.

Objectives of the intervention

Starting in 2015, funded and with technical advice from HATD, the Aid Organization for Refugees and Asylum Seekers in Israel (ASSAF) and the Israel AIDS Task Force (IATF) implemented a joint project serving refugees and asylum seekers (RAS) living with HIV as well as the general RAS population. The project's goals were, first, to promote rights and services for RAS living with HIV, equal to the rights and services enjoyed by Israelis in a similar situation, and second, to educate the RAS public about HIV and HIV prevention. The project accomplished this by: 1) training two community members as HIV consultants; 2) educating the RAS communities on HIV prevention, rights, and services available; 3) providing case management for RAS living with HIV and their families; and 4) advocating for RAS rights and policy changes at the governmental level. This chapter reports on the intervention, detailing its successes and challenges both from a measurement and policy/political point of view.

Aid Organization for Refugees and Asylum Seekers in Israel (ASSAF)

ASSAF promotes the welfare and rights of RAS by providing advocacy services and psychosocial support for asylum seekers at the individual and community levels while engaging in macro-level advocacy to change public discourse and official Israeli policy.[16] Since 2007, ASSAF has been the central Israeli organization offering psychosocial support and programs for the most vulnerable RAS, including:

- survivors of torture and human trafficking,
- women who suffer from domestic violence,
- individuals with physical and mental disabilities,
- HIV carriers and AIDS patients, and
- youths aged 9–19

Israel AIDS Task Force (IATF[17])

IATF was founded in 1985, at the start of the AIDS epidemic, with the mission to stop the spread of the AIDS epidemic in Israel and to protect and promote the rights, interests, quality of life, and life expectancy of people living with HIV.

Brief year by year description of IATF/ASSAF activities and accomplishments for the four years of the initiative

In year I

Working with RAS community workers, the IATF/ASSAF community health workers (CHW) became increasingly known in the RAS community as HIV knowledge experts and go-to people to obtain needed services. RAS call the CHWs to ask HIV-related questions. For example, some have asked if they can get infected after performing oral sex. Twenty workshops, including those for women, were conducted in the first year, with 403 people attending. The evaluation report was based on IATF's work, using evaluation questionnaires that were fielded before and after educational workshops providing information about, and tools to deal with HIV/AIDS, stigma, and safe sex. Unfortunately, only 36 of the 403 returned questionnaires. For example, in the IATF visit to Holot, where 158 participated in IATF workshops, no one filled out the questionnaire, as IATF staff were not allowed to bring them into the facility. In other workshops, participants were reluctant to fill them out. Thus, this chapter does not include any summary of the questionnaire results.

IATF also successfully lobbied the Israeli government for the inception of appropriate medication treatment for HIV-positive RAS who were held in Holot detention center. The IATF managed to persuade the Israeli Ministry of Health to continue their treatment once they were released from Holot. ASSAF provided counseling to 28 HIV-positive RAS. Since the coordinators are exposed to disturbing content that can take an emotional toll on them and the two community consultants, ASSAF and IATF's coordinator and the two community consultants receive outside support provided by two certified psychologists. IATF Israeli volunteers living with HIV consisted mainly of gay men who do not speak Tigrinya, a language spoken in Eritrea and Ethiopia. The RAS community found it difficult to open themselves to a person so different from their culture.

In year 2

Activities

ASSAF and IATF spent a considerable amount of time at the beginning of year 2 refining the questionnaires and adopting new strategies to obtain maximum reliability and validity for questionnaire completion. IATF conducted 12 workshops with 450 participants. Of these, 191 were tested (at IATF's testing center/mobile clinic). IATF staff accompanied more than 20 HIV-positive people for treatment during this time. A week's activities typically included:

- Meeting with HIV-positive RAS who are not fully aware of their needs and treatment options.
- Case management and support for beneficiaries on an as-needed basis, which includes accompanying people to appointments (for example, to hospitals and outpatient medical centers and AIDS centers, the Center for Tuberculosis, UNHCR, Physicians for Human Rights-Israel, or PHRI), speaking with beneficiaries on the phone, conducting meetings in the community, doing intakes and periodic psychosocial evaluations with the ASSAF psychosocial counselor, or helping with translations for communication with the beneficiaries.
- Promoting the interests of HIV-positive RAS within the Israeli Ministry of Health (MoH).
- Conducting workshops, both preplanned and spontaneous, in main gathering areas and recreational places of the RAS community.

Joint efforts between ASSAF and IATF

- Together, these organizations produced a short YouTube video about HIV, with RAS community-related topics. Within twenty-four hours it received 35,000 views and 179 likes. A week later, it reported more than 69,300 views, 320 likes, and 485 shares.

- IATF and ASSAF conducted three educational workshops for mothers and the staff teaching kindergarten. Some of the women even took condoms and asked them to give more workshops.

IATF

- Tel Hashomer Hospital, a major hospital in Tel Aviv, began offering medical tests for pregnant HIV-positive RAS.
- Reached out to Holot detention center and conducted four educational workshops with 343 participants. IATF also conducted a testing day, with 56 people coming to the IATF mobile unit.
- An HIV-positive asylum seeker reached out to IATF with a CD4 count of 0, meaning that the AIDS was completely uncontrolled. In less than a week IATF was able to refer her to the community program, and she began to receive appropriate medication.

ASSAF

- Psychosocial support was given to 45 RAS throughout the year; 28 RAS are currently in the project. A total of 68 evaluations with 36 clients (each of whom completed between one to four evaluations) were carried out in the project, with more than 16 evaluations done in the second year.

Results of year 2 evaluation of workshops

In the second year, after a complete restructuring of the questionnaires, IATF distributed questionnaires in eight workshops. In total, 184 participants answered the questionnaires. Of these, 22 were women in two groups. IATF also obtained data from four of the groups (one group of women) for post-workshop questionnaires with 33 respondents. All of the participants were of Eritrean descent.

Overall well-being

Participants reported an overall small increase in well-being from the time of their first evaluation to the time of their last. Of note, women and victims of torture experienced greater increases in well-being than their counterparts.

Blame

Across subgroups, the participants experienced a slight decrease in the amount of blame they felt. Women and victims of torture reported the greatest negative change, indicating that their feelings of blame had been alleviated somewhat over the course of this project.

Stigma

On average, participants reported a slight decrease over time in the degree of stigma they experienced in their daily lives within the community. At the start of the project, all participants stated that they faced a high level of stigma in the community. Over time, women and victims of torture reported the greatest change in the level of stigma they felt, with results indicating that they feel less stigmatized now than they did when they began participating in the project.

Perceptions of social support

Sense of support was measured in order to understand if the participants felt they could be supported by ASSAF or from within their own community. Across all subgroups of participants, there was a significant increase in the sense of support, with women and victims of torture reporting the greatest increase in perceptions of social support. Participants reported "ASSAF," "social worker," "doctor," "church," and "friend" as people they could count on for social support.

Interpretation of year 2 results

By the end of year 2, women experienced an increase in physical and emotional well-being, and a significant decrease in both self-blame about the infection and feeling of stigma. Women also showed a sizable increase in perceptions of social support. Although men did not demonstrate improvement in well-being, they did not experience a deterioration in emotional well-being. Like the women, they reported a decrease in self-blame and stigma, as well as a considerable increase in perception of social support. At the beginning of the program, when naming their sources of social support, many participants named no one. By the end, many named ASSAF's social worker as a source of social support. This was especially true of men, who are often with-out families, unlike women, many of whom benefited from familial relationships. Having social support proved extremely valuable.

Previous research shows the detrimental effects of torture: depres-sion, anxiety, self-helplessness, impaired memory and concentration, fear of intimacy, and somatic symptoms.[18] It is therefore not surprising that the victims of torture (VOT) reported lower cognitive, emotional, and overall well-being. Comparisons with participants who were not victims of torture indicate that the project is especially helpful to clients who are coping with traumas and hardships as a result of tor-ture. Many VOT contracted HIV as a result of sexual violence per-petrated against them, and they bear heavy burdens of subsequent self-blame and stigma. Over time in the program, VOT showed a slight decrease in self-blame and a sizable decrease in stigma, as well as a substantial increase in perceptions of social support. These were important, positive results in the most vulnerable clients. The psy-chosocial work targeting and countering self-blame and stigma about HIV also addressed the stigma surrounding torture and violence.

Not receiving medication can, not surprisingly, have a significant physical and psychological impact on an individual. However, the medication of asylum seekers who receive it is often second-generation medication, meaning that it may be less effective. The government program provides only this type of medication, as it is cheaper than first-line medication. As a result, some participants reported feeling poorly and having bad side effects shortly after taking medications. The results of the analysis concerning medication varied wildly and were, not surprisingly, very inconsistent.

As was true throughout this initiative, ASSAF and IATF faced several challenges in obtaining data. Some of the asylum seekers cannot read or write and thus sometimes show reluctance to fill out the questionnaire, in order not to expose themselves to their peers. Moreover, some of them simply did not wish to fill out the question-naires, regardless of their literacy status. This is partly because they felt uncomfortable answering questions relating to sex and their sex-ual habits (e.g., condom use). Those who filled out the questionnaire were mostly the more educated participants in workshops, who come from a stronger socioeconomic background in their home country. Trying to learn from year 1, IATF conducted a verbal questionnaire for post-workshop evaluation. Even so, IATF still found it difficult to get in contact with many of the participants to obtain answers to this verbal, over the phone, questionnaire.

In year 3

ASSAF continued its counseling and community work in the last year of the program. As mentioned above, for a twenty-four-hour period in 2018, the Israeli government negotiated an agreement with the UNHCR to give refugee status to many RAS in return for the UNHCR resettling the remainder in third countries. After intense right-wing pushback, the conservative government of Benjamin Netanyahu pressed to have the entire RAS community deported to different African countries (with payment to these countries of a substantial sum per RAS). In the third year, the IATF focused on the political and legal fight against this deportation program. HATD raised additional funds via a crowd funding campaign to support the fight.

Examples of this struggle

An HIV patient received a pre-deportation hearing but refused to reveal the fact that he was HIV-positive to the Ministry of Interior (he feared that MoI would not keep the medical information confidential, and IATF was unsuccessful in its efforts to convince him otherwise). Nevertheless, with the assistance of the Refugee Rights Clinic, his deportation was canceled without revealing his status, as his wife had just given birth, and fathers of children are excluded from deportation at this stage.

Another HIV patient failed to renew his visa for a long time due to severe physical and emotional problems (he had been diagnosed several months before with a low CD4 count, meaning that the disease was not well controlled). The IATF provided him with a letter explaining the situation and he managed to renew his visa without being summoned to a pre-deportation hearing.

With the active involvement of IATF and additional fund-raising support from HATD, the High Court of Justice issued a temporary order freezing the deportation process to Rwanda until the state responded to the petitions filed against deportation. The government eventually gave up on the deportation, but it has made life increasingly difficult for the remaining RAS community.

In year 4, the last year of the program

In 2018–19, the project was not operated in conjunction with IATF. The final evaluation report was based on individual psychosocial evaluations of participants in the program. These consisted of questionnaires administered verbally by the social worker managing the client's case or by a community health worker in the program acting as a linguistic and cultural interpreter (in Tigrinya, Arabic, Amharic, English, and Hebrew) to facilitate communication. Psychosocial evaluations were administered every few months. For a more detailed description of the revisions, please see the section "Measures."

Sample

At the end of the last year of the project, 48 asylum seekers living with HIV/AIDS in Israel, 25 males and 23 females (from ages 25 to 58 years, though for various reasons, such as lack of documentation, the exact age of many asylum seekers is not known), completed psychosocial evaluations. Most of the participants were from Eritrea and Sudan, the rest from other African countries. Whereas 108 psychosocial evaluations were completed in total by 48 individuals, 34 individuals completed more than one evaluation (either two, three, or four evaluations). In order to evaluate change over time, for the purpose of this chapter, the data analyzed includes only those participants who completed more than one evaluation. The data compares the changes in their results over time, from the first psychosocial evaluation, the second, the third, and, for whom it is relevant, the fourth psychosocial evaluation.

Measures

The evaluation consisted of a two-part survey, covering well-being and stigma, based on a Likert scale (questionnaire available on request). Each participant was asked to fill out the survey during their intake and then ideally every three to four months. In reality, this was not realistic for every participant, for several reasons: 1) some clients are so vulnerable (emotionally or physically) that answering the evaluation questionnaire would have triggered their post-traumatic stress disorder (PTSD), doing more harm than good; 2) while some clients had completed the first evaluation questionnaire, their treatment did not continue on a regular basis, foreclosing the opportunity to fill out a second evaluation; 3) other clients were not interested in completing the evaluation questionnaire, and ASSAF staff respected their request. Additionally, the use of the Likert scale presented obstacles; many participants found it difficult to use numbers to assess their feelings and preferred to answer the questions verbally. This created a further challenge, as assigning a number depending on a verbal response left room for interpretation and inconsistencies between administrators of the evaluation. ASSAF staff added an open-ended question to learn more about whom participants turned to when they needed support.

The evaluation provided more than measures of assessment. It also enabled the clients to bring up critical issues they confronted that would not always come up otherwise in treatment. The evaluation was always done by the social worker, sometimes with the help of a community health worker. The questions addressed four different areas of well-being (physical, emotional, cognitive, and overall), as well as self-blame, stigma, and perception of social support.

Well-being was measured through four different areas: physical, emotional, cognitive, and overall well-being. Questions were taken from Medical Outcomes Study (MOS)-HIV, World Health Organization Quality of Life (WHO QOL)-HIV, and the Coping Self-Efficacy Scale.[19] Questions were chosen based on relevance and cultural appropriateness. In order to measure social support and community and internal stigma, questions were taken from HIV Related Stigma Measure and HIV Stigma Scale. Again, questions were chosen for their relevance and cultural appropriateness. Community and internal stigma were measured.

Results

The results of the analysis of the sample are summarized below. It is important to note that the results are only for the sample of participants who filled two evaluations or more (29 participants).

Physical well-being

Questions focused on physical well-being were designed to measure the amount of physical pain that a person performed on a daily basis. Most reported increased well-being and decreased pain.

Emotional well-being

Participants who received HIV medication reported an increase in their emotional well-being, whereas participants who did not receive HIV medication reported minimal change in their emotional well-being. Men showed an increase in emotional well-being between the first and second psychosocial evaluation. Women, on the other hand, showed an increase in emotional well-being between the second and third psychosocial evaluation. Participants who were not survivors of torture in Sinai reported an increase in emotional well-being, while those who were survivors of torture in Sinai did not show strong changes over time. The participants did not report a significant change in cognitive well-being over the evaluations. Most participants experienced a decrease in self-blame and stigma. Finally, the participants reported a marginally increased sense of support over time, specifically, from friends and the community.

Discussion and concluding comments

In the last year reported in this chapter, RAS served by ASSAF reported a marginal increase in well-being over time. In year 4, women living with HIV demonstrated lower levels of emotional well-being compared with their male counterparts. This is in line with studies that suggest that women living with HIV experience a lower quality of life, fewer supports, and more depression than men living with HIV.[20] However, across the evaluations, both men and women reported an increase in emotional well-being, though the increase was greater for women.

Limitations of these questionnaires need to be acknowledged. All variables were measured by self-report instruments, which may have caused bias. The Likert scale caused some difficulties for many participants. The evaluation was further limited by the sample size. Some individuals who had completed a first evaluation did not continue with the program, for various reasons.

The results must be looked at in light of the overall situation confronting the RAS in Israel, which has worsened since 2019. Other factors external to the program are at play—specifically, lack of access to quality health care, welfare, and rights—and continue to play a detrimental role for this most vulnerable group. Israeli policy has had a major detrimental effect on the well-being of RAS living with HIV. ASSAF staff has observed a significant decline in the mental state of all clients. Staff witnessed increased numbers of clients dealing with PTSD and depression. After a long stay in Israel, many of ASSAF's clients speak of decreased hope for the future.

As a result of Israel's extreme discriminatory policy, the asylum seekers' situation in Israel has not improved. Israel has failed to consider and examine asylum applications for more than twelve years and has left the RAS community with limited access to health and social services, denial of social security and work permits, and a law that further penalizes the RAS.[21] Such policy and practice explicitly aim to pressure them to leave Israel despite their protected status. Tragically, the most vulnerable asylum seekers are most affected by Israeli policy: people with disabilities and chronic health conditions, women and children, street dwellers, and victims of torture. They are also the least likely to be accepted by a third country in either Europe or North America.

Postscript: a personal note

Returning to the conundrum highlighted at the beginning of this chapter, the HATD Board of Directors continues to support humanitarian efforts to improve the lives of the most vulnerable RAS population. This will continue despite the fact that the RAS are neither Israeli nor Palestinian. We hope that ongoing purely humanitarian support of this harshly treated population will not only improve the health of a few but also shine a light on Israel's terrible human rights record with respect to these individuals, many of whom fled genocidal wars. This is especially unfortunate considering the tragic history of many of Israel's present inhabitants, who fled another genocidal regime, that of Nazi Germany.

Appendix: Client and community health worker stories

With the help of ASSAF, an HIV-positive husband brings his wife into treatment

N is an asylum seeker from Eritrea, married with three children. In 2015, he was tested for HIV and discovered he is positive but told no one. In 2018, his health deteriorated; he became sick with tuberculosis and AIDS and was hospitalized for a long period. He began receiving HIV medicine but continued to keep his illness a secret from his wife. After N joined the project in ASSAF and developed a close relationship of trust with the social worker, he expressed the concern that he had infected his wife. He said he wanted to tell her the truth but did not know how. With the support of the social worker, N told his wife and brought her to IATF to be tested. Within minutes the test came back positive. Even though the couple was prepared for the result, it was difficult for them to hear. This has created a breach of trust between the couple, especially given their fears about their children's health. The project staff has continued to support the family through this crisis. It is fortunate that the wife discovered her condition before it deteriorated and led to hospitalization, as often happens. She may be eligible for the HAART program and will do a CD4 test soon. She was also immediately integrated into the project, for close psychosocial support and ongoing guidance.

ASSAF finds treatment and housing for an HIV-positive female

L is an asylum seeker from South Africa, HIV carrier, mother of five children, and nine months pregnant. She came to Israel in October 2016, found a female roommate, and occasionally worked as a janitor. As her pregnancy progressed, she could not work as much; as a result, her income decreased and she found herself homeless. With ASSAF's mediation, she entered a women's shelter. ASSAF's social worker looked for an alternative place of residence for L once she gave birth, contacting shelters, churches, and the Tel Aviv municipality. All rejected the woman. Then ASSAF found a Christian organization in Jerusalem that has an apartment, with meals and assistance for the baby. ASSAF continued to work with the woman after she gave birth.

ASSAF provides treatment and employment for an HIV-positive female

M is a single mother of a three-year-old girl, who was born in Israel, and a nine-year-old son, who was born in Eritrea and is still there. M was kidnapped in Sinai and held there as a sex slave for three months. When she was pregnant with her daughter, she discovered that she had contracted HIV as a result of her rape in the Sinai. M suffered severe violence from the father of her daughter, who accused her of infecting him with HIV. After her partner left her, she engaged in prostitution for a period of time in order to support herself and her daughter.

M suffered severe stigma in the RAS community when her friend told her secret and her HIV status became known. Her state— penniless, a victim of domestic violence, working in prostitution, and isolated from her community—left her severely depressed. Because of her mental state, she would leave her daughter in the nursery for days without coming to pick her up. After ASSAF and IATF worked with M for a long time, her mental state improved. She is no longer secretive and isolated and is much more open and sharing. M has been receiving medical treatment for the last six months; she has quit prostitution and has steady employment.

M has a regular partner, whom she had not told about her HIV status. After ASSAF's intervention, receiving treatment for some time, and many discussions on the subject, M told her partner about her status. M also received humanitarian assistance from ASSAF for six months and food donations during the difficult times. M began to learn English and ASSAF submitted her application to the United Nations for resettlement.

ASSAF finds treatment for an HIV-positive couple

An ASSAF social worker has been accompanying a family that was referred to ASSAF by another beneficiary of the program. The family is composed of a husband (D) and wife (L), aged 31, and two children, aged 4 and 6. Asylum seekers from Eritrea, they met in a refugee camp in Sudan. Before L arrived in the refugee camp, she was abducted and imprisoned in Sudan, where she was raped on a daily basis until she managed to escape. On their way to Israel the couple was kidnapped by Bedouins in Sinai, and because they could not pay ransom they were kept captive for four months, during which time they were severely abused physically and sexually. After they were released, they entered Israel, and within a short period each began to work. Both of their sons were born in Israel. In her ninth month of pregnancy, L discovered that she was HIV-positive; D was tested as well and also found to be positive. L received treatment for six months after the birth of her first son, and then again in her second pregnancy. But since then neither L nor D has received medicine. About nine months ago, D was admitted to the hospital and began receiving medicine under the Ministry of Health's plan. A short time later, L also began to receive treatment.

However, both developed severe drug reactions (the drugs included in the program are old-generation drugs). Both suffer from depression, insomnia, and dizziness. L also suffers from disorientation and anemia, due to the medication. The couple is in great distress about their physical and mental health; both are unable to work regularly for long and subsequently have many financial difficulties. The ASSAF CHW is in constant contact with the doctor who is treating the couple, and the doctor submitted a request for a change in their medicines. In the month of August, L tried to commit suicide. She asked D to take the children to the park and while they were out drank bleach. Luckily, her friend (the same friend who referred them to ASSAF) came to visit her. She found L only moments after she had attempted suicide. With amazing resourcefulness, she made L drink milk, which caused L to vomit. She called an ambulance and then called the ASSAF CHW; the latter went to the hospital and called D, who was seriously shaken up by the turn of events. L was hospitalized for one night and then released. In the meantime, the Ministry of Health approved dispensing the new generation of drugs (but only after initially refusing and the doctor appealed the decision). This story is just one in a series of many in which we bear witness to the administration of an older class of drugs with severe side effects to the RAS HIV community, which carries serious implications for the patients' physical and mental health conditions. This issue—the nature and selection of drugs used in the national program—is widespread, and we have included it in the ASSAF advocacy program.

Disappearance of patients and ASSAF'S inability to locate them

S is an asylum seeker from Eritrea, a single mother of a one-and-a-half-year-old (and two children aged 8 and 12 in Eritrea). S is HIV-positive and a survivor of domestic violence. It is suspected that she works in prostitution. She is not eligible for drug treatment through the National Health Ministry's program because the CD4 count, a measure of HIV activity, count is too high. After many deliberations, ASSAF's staff decided to try and obtain medical treatment for S. Her doctor was very cooperative; he referred her for a viral load test and CD4 count and enrolled her in the treatment program. ASSAF's intention was to raise S's CD4 using medicine IATF receives as donations and then have her moved to the program. Unfortunately, S did not come in to do the viral load test, and ASSAF staff has been unable to contact her. Since then her telephone has been disconnected and her son has been removed from nursery school. ASSAF staff even attempted to visit her at her house, without any luck.

ASSAF staff continue to look and hope to find her soon and then be able to give an encouraging update to the story.

An Eritrean community worker for ASSAF

I was born in Awhne, a village located in South Eastern Eritrea, in 10/06/1980. I grew up with my family full of love, affection, and good treatment by my parents, grandparents, and other fellow family members. The economy of my family was relying on agriculture and producing of some domestic animals. I actively participated in helping my family from my childhood as much as I can. When my age reached to education, I started school in my village Awhne and learned until grade five. After I completed elementary school I transferred to the nearby town of Adikeih in order to continue junior and high school levels. Though I have been faced with big problems to complete my high school due to distance of school, by hard working of me and my family, I successfully finished in the year 2000. I scored good results in the national examination and joined the University of Asmara in September 2000. I graduated from the university in the field of Sociology and Social Work in July 16, 2004. After I graduated the government assigned me to the Ministry of Labor and Human Welfare in the labor department as employment promoter as part of my national service. I worked in the Ministry for eight years.

Since I protested different labor laws and policies of the Ministry, I was referred to Adi Abeito detention center for questioning by national security. I didn't feel secure and safe in my home country, since many were disappeared, jailed in secretive detentions without been seen by the court of law for years. I crossed to Sudan by foot on 04/04/2012 illegally and entered Shegerab refugee camp located in the Eastern Sudan. I found the place was insecure and risky due to high human trafficking, and some forced deportation was happened by the Sudan's government because of the good diplomatic ties of the two dictators. I thought that the only safe place to stay is Israel and decided to travel to Israel. After one month, terrible and harsh journey through the Sahara Desert and danger of human trafficking in Sinai, I arrived in Israel on 15/05/2012.

In Israel, I have been involved in different activities with different humanitarian organizations like Amnesty International Israel, ARDC, and Eritrean Community Women center as volunteer. Eritrean Community Women Center is the only grassroot NGO run by the women asylum seekers. I helped the center for one year as a volunteer in translating different fliers, booklets and filling refugee status determination forms (RSD). I also worked with Amnesty in translating monthly community updates and refugee connected developments.

Notes

1 United Nations High Commission on Refugees (2011) *Convention and Protocol Relating to the Status of Refugees.* Available at https://www.unhcr.org/3b66c2aa10. Accessed: June 7, 2020, p. 3.
2 Available at https://www.hias.org/where/israel. Accessed: June 7, 2020.

3   Reuters (2018) Israel's Netanyahu puts African migrant deal with UNHCR on hold. Reuters. Available at: https://www.reuters.com/article/us-israel-migrants-netanyahu-idUSKCN1H91TL Accessed: June 27, 2020.

4   Weitz, G., Glazer, W. (2020) How Israel tried to dump African refugees in blood-drenched dictatorships. *Haaretz.* Available at: https://www.haaretz.com/israel-news/.premium.MAGAZINE-how-israel-tried-to-dump-african-refugees-in-blood-drenched-dictatorships-1.9398948. Accessed: February 2021.

5   Berman, Y. (2016) The Labyrinth: migration, status and human rights. pp. 50–51. Available at: https://law.acri.org.il/en/2016/01/05/the-labrynth-migration-status-and-human-rights/. Accessed: February 2021.

6   Vanable, PA., Carey, MP., Blair, DC., et al. (2006) Impact of HIV-related stigma on health behaviors and psychological adjustment among HIV-positive men and women. *AIDS Behav.* 10(5), pp: 473-482.

7   Gordillo, V., Fekete, E., Platteau, T., et al. (2009). Emotional support and gender in people living with HIV: Effects on psychological well-being. *Journal of Behavioral Medicine.* 32(6), pp: 523–531.

8   Cruess, D., Evans, D., Repetto, M., et al. (2003). Prevalence, diagnosis, and pharmacological treatment of mood disorders in HIV disease. *Biological Psychiatry.* 54 (3) pp: 307–316.

9   Bing, EG., Burnam, MA., Longshore, D., et al. (2001) Psychiatric disorders and drug use among human immunodeficiency virus-infected adults in the United States. *Arch Gen Psychiatry.* 58(8), pp: 721-728.

10 Leserman, J. (2008) Role of depression, stress, and trauma in HIV disease progression. *Psychosom Med.* 70(5), pp: 539-545.

11 Gonzalez. JS., Penedo, FJ., Antoni, MH., et al. (2004) Social support, positive states of mind, and HIV treatment adherence in men and women living with HIV/AIDS. *Health Psychol.* 23(4), pp: 413-418.

12 Deichert, NT., Fekete, EM., Boarts, JM., et al. (2008) Emotional support and affect: associations with health behaviors and active coping efforts in men living with HIV. *AIDS and Behavior.* 12(1), pp: 139–145.

13 Safren, SA., Radomsky, AS., Otto, MW., et al. (2002) Predictors of psychological well-being in a diverse sample of HIV-positive patients receiving highly active antiretroviral therapy. *Psychosomatics.* 43(6), pp: 478–485.

14 Catz, S.L, Gore-Felton, C., McClure, JB. (2002) Psychological distress among minority and low-income women living with HIV. *Behavioral Medicine* (Washington, D.C.). 28(2), pp: 53–60.

15 Gitelson, B. Inside Sinai's Torture Camps. (2012) *The Atlantic.* Available at: https://www.theatlantic.com/international/archive/2012/11/inside-sinais-torture-camps/265204/ Accessed: June 7, 2020.

16 See http://assaf.org.il/en/node/2.

17 See https://www.aidsisrael.org.il/article/israel-aids-task-force.

18 Gorman, W. (2001). Refugee survivors of torture: Trauma and treatment. *Professional Psychology: Research and Practice* 200L. 32 (5), pp: 443–451.

19 Shahriar, J., Delate, T., Hays, R. D., et al. (2003). Commentary on using the SF-36 or MOS-HIV in studies of persons with HIV disease. *Health and Quality of Life Outcomes, 1* (25), pp: 1–7. Available at https://www.ncbi.nlm.nih.gov/pmc/articles/PMC183842/pdf/1477–7525–1–25.pdf; Accessed: June 13, 2020; WHO-QOL HIV https://www.who.int/mental_health/media/en/557.pdf Accessed: June 13, 2020; Coping Self-Efficacy Scale https://prevention.ucsf.edu/research-project/coping-self-efficacy-scale-scoring. Accessed: June 13, 2020.

20 Cederfjäll, C., Langius-Eklöf, A., Lidman, K., et al. (2001) Gender differ-
    ences in perceived health-related quality of life among patients with HIV
    infection. *AIDS Patient Care and STDs* 15 (1), pp: 31–39. Available at https://
    home.liebertpub.com/publications/aids-patient-care-and-stds/1. Accessed:
    June 13, 2020.
21 Available   at   https://www.haaretz.com/israel-news/.premium-israel-s-
    top-court-strikes-down-law-requiring-asylum-seekers-to-deposit-20-of-
    wages-1.8794068. Accessed: February 2020. Note just recently during the
    COVID-19 crisis the Israeli Supreme Court declared the law invalid. It
    remains to be seen if the Israeli government tries other ways of garnishing
    RAS wages.

Chapter 6

Beterem

Grandmothers for social change in an Arab town in Northern Israel

Gali Malkin, Elad Calif, Daniela Orr and
Norbert Goldfield

Introduction

This initiative examined the effectiveness of a home visit intervention program consisting of local senior women providing an evidence-based child safety intervention in a low-income Israeli Arab community. Injury is the leading cause of death in children and young adults. According to the Centers for Disease Control and Prevention, approximately 12,000 children and young adults, aged 1 to 19 years, die from unintentional injuries in the United States each year.[1] Researchers and policymakers have extensively examined interventions to decrease avoidable childhood accidents at home and concluded that they generally have had an impact. Since 1990, for example, total injury mortality among children under 15 years of age at home has declined by more than two-thirds in Germany.[2] Reviews of randomized and non-randomized trials and interventions published since 2010 have increased the fund of information.[3] The interventions they describe have occurred in a variety of settings, including health care institutions, homes, and schools.[4] Most of these trials have discerned a positive effect of these interventions on salient outcomes, such as knowledge,[5] visits to a health care professional,[6] and risks and rates of traumatic injuries.[7]

Low-income and/or ethnic minority children are the groups most at risk for home childhood accidents.[8] Studies from around the world have shown an inverse relation between poverty and childhood injury, morbidity and mortality. Compared with children from well-off families, children from low-income families have higher rates of morbidity and mortality of traffic accidents, fires, falls, and drownings and an increased risk of hospitalization from play injuries.[9]

Focusing on the Israeli context, Israeli Arab children are at higher risk for unintentional injuries compared with their Jewish counterparts.[10] Although Arabs make up a fifth of the population and their children constitute 26% of all those under age 18, 50% of children who die from unintentional injuries are Arabs.[11] These gaps between the two population groups have persisted and continue to grow. Moreover, differences between Israeli Arabs and Jews increase with the severity of the injury.[12] The HATD-funded intervention featured here was carried out to address these gaps. It took place in Tur'an, a local council in the Northern District of Israel in which Israeli Arab citizens predominate. We examined the effectiveness of a home visits initiative, conducted among Israeli Arab families and targeted at improving their overall house safety.

A significant aspect of the intervention pertains to the central role played by senior citizens, specifically grandmothers, in this community. Researchers have pointed to the importance of senior citizens in assuming functions that the government and private sector have either abandoned or never assumed.[13] In this initiative, the intervention was undertaken by grandmothers of the community, who received safety training and performed the home visits—the first intervention to employ a child safety intervention program involving senior women as change agents. The work of the grandmothers included activities such as identifying life-endangering safety hazards, providing safety guidance to children, and supplying a safety accessories kit.

Method

Participating organizations

Three organizations were involved in the implementation of this initiative. Beterem is a nonprofit organization that aims to promote child safety and to create a safer environment for children in Israel. It has been a Safe Kids Worldwide member since 2001. The Tur'an Community Center is a nationally-supported government center delivering local community services. Such community centers exist in many "recognized" (meaning that the town receives government services such as electricity, running water, and bus services) Israeli towns and villages. Healing Across the Divides also participated.

Beterem was the overall implementer, primarily responsible for the initiative. It worked through the Tur'an Community Center to recruit the seniors leading the intervention. Healing Across the Divides furnished funding as well as expertise in research design, literature review, and community-based change.

Participants

A total of 159 Arab families living in the Northern District of Israel participated in the intervention: 67 families participated in the first wave of the intervention (in the years 2015–16), 69 families in the second wave (in the year 2017), and 23 families in the third wave (in the year 2018). The families were recruited via trained instructors—senior women residing in the local community who volunteered to participate in a child safety intervention initiative and received training on child safety. The instructors asked eligible women from their community to take part in a program aimed to improve child safety. Table 6.1 summarizes the socio-demographic characteristics of the participating families.

Table 6.1 Socio-demographic characteristics of the participants

Variables	First wave (n=67)	Second wave (n=69)	Third wave (n=23)
Educational level of mother			
Less than 12 years	3 (4%)	4 (6%)	0
12 years (high school)	18 (27%)	25 (36%)	8 (35%)
More than 12 years	46 (69%)	40 (58%)	15 (65%)
Educational level of father			
Less than 12 years	2 (3%)	11 (16%)	2 (9%)
12 years (high school)	24 (36%)	31 (46%)	10 (43%)
More than 12 years	40 (61%)	26 (38%)	11 (48%)
Number of children under 18 years			
0	30 (45%)	16 (23%)	11 (48%)
1	9 (13%)	9 (13%)	3 (13%)
2	13 (19%)	18 (26%)	4 (17%)
3	9 (13%)	19 (28%)	1 (4%)
4 +	6 (9%)	7 (10%)	4 (17%)
	Mean (SD)	Mean (SD)	Mean (SD)
Age of mother	37.46 (11.40)	37.01 (8.79)	34.95 (9.37)
Age of father	41.46 (9.70)	42.14 (8.46)	38.85 (9.04)

Intervention

"Home visits" is an intervention program that takes place in the homes of women from the community. The program used an evidence-based checklist and included identifying life-threatening safety hazards and deficiencies, transmitting information on child safety, supplying practical tools and accessories for intervention, and providing information about additional safety accessories necessary for keeping children safe at home and in the yard.

For each of the participating families, the volunteering instructor was asked to make two home visits, spaced about three months apart. In this way it was possible to ascertain whether the level of home safety had improved in response to the initiative, both in terms of making changes in the home to adapt it for children and in adopting safety practices to prevent injuries.

Each home visit session began with a brief phone call made by the instructors to eligible mothers, in which the instructor introduced herself and asked to schedule a counseling meeting on child safety with the mother. It was explained that the meeting would be held in the family home. After receiving the mother's approval and scheduling the date, the instructor carried out the first visit. Each visit was held in a standard format, consisting of (a) a self-introduction and a brief description of the visit, explaining that it would include filling out a safety checklist to locate potential safety hazards across the house. On receiving the mother's consent, each instructor moved to the next phase, in which (b) the rationale for conducting the home visit was explained. The instructor described briefly each child safety problem, along with its scope and consequences. Next, the instructor (c) reviewed practical tools available to improve child safety, such as modifying the physical environment of the house and adopting safety habits. The instructor then (d) introduced the checklist questionnaire, and the tour of the house began. The instructor and the mother examined each room according to the format prescribed by the questionnaire. The instructor completed the questionnaire and, based on the findings, she gave (e) recommendations to fix potential hazards that were observed in the visit. At the final stage (f), the instructor handed out a safety kit containing several safety accessories (cabinet fasteners, electrical outlet covers, anti-slip stickers for the bathroom, and door anti-slammers) and a summary sheet with brief information messages on child safety.

The second home visit session, carried out three to six months following the first visit, examined whether improvements in the overall house safety levels were evident, based on the recommendations that were delivered in the first visit. In the second visit, the same checklist questionnaire was again filled out by the instructor. Overall, the intervention was implemented across three years: the first wave of the intervention was held between October 2015 and December 2016, the second wave between May and September 2017, and the third wave between January 2018 and December 2018.

The checklist questionnaire

The checklist, adapted from previous work, includes general background questions and questions aimed to trace necessary changes needed to improve child safety.[14] It covers ten major categories: the kitchen cooking area, the kitchen eating area, storage and use of detergents, medication and pesticides, electricity, and the like. For each category, several questions specify the potential hazard or change to be made. For example: "when the children (0–4) eat, Are they under the supervision of an adult?"; "Are the detergents kept in a place that is high up or locked?"; and "Is there a safety circuit breaker at home?" Three answer options are offered for each of these items: "yes" (for a safe situation); "no" (for an unsafe situation); and "irrelevant" (if the object in question is absent from the house). Overall, the checklist consists of 30 items.

Analysis

In order to determine whether there was a change in household safety levels between the first and second visits, the total score for each household on each visit was calculated. Each item marked "yes," indicating a safe situation, was coded as 1, while the unsafe situation was coded as 0. Scores for all items were summarized and mean scores for each house in each visit calculated. The primary outcome measure was the difference between the two home visits' mean scores. Additionally, the implementation of positive changes (that is, items that changed from "no" to "yes" in the second visit) and the presence of negative changes (that is, items that changed from "yes" to "no" in the second visit) were examined.

Results

Positive changes between the first and second visit

Table 6.2 presents the aggregate number of positive changes (items that changed from "no" in the first visit to "yes" in the second visit) in each year of the intervention. It is evident that across all three waves, at least one positive change was observed in the vast majority of the households.

The data reveals that the most common positive change, made in 67%–87% of the households during the three years of the program, was "use of accessories to prevent door slamming." (This accessory was handed out by the instructors in the first visit.) Additional positive changes that featured prominently were: the installation of window bars or restricting window openings, fixing closets and cabinets to the wall, installing a fence separating a parking area from the children's play area, and keeping detergents in a high or locked place.

Negative changes between the first and second visit

The number of items that changed from "yes" in the first visit to "no" in the second visit was also reviewed. The results are described

Table 6.2 Number of positive changes between first and second visit

Number of changes made	First year (n=67)		Second year (n=69)		Third year (n=23)	
	Number of households	%	Number of households	%	Number of households	%
No changes	7	10.4%	0		1	4.3%
1–2 changes	30	44.8%	29	42.0%	5	21.7%
3–4 changes	22	32.8%	22	31.9%	7	30.4%
5 or more changes	8	12.0%	18	26.1%	10	43.4%
Mean (SD)		2.33 (1.69)		3.59 (2.66)		4.47 (3.16)

Table 6.3 Number of negative changes between first and second visit

Number of changes made	First year (n=67)		Second year (n=69)		Third year (n=23)	
	Number of household	%	Number of households	%	Number of households	%
No changes	28	41.8%	41	59.4%	20	87.0%
1–2 changes	30	44.8%	27	39.1%	2	8.7%
3–4 changes	8	12.0%	1	1.4%	1	4.3%
5 or more changes	1	1.5%	0		0	
Mean (SD)	1.13	(1.33)	0.61 (0.86)		0.21 (0.67)	

in Table 6.3. Across all three years of the intervention, most of the cases in the negative changes distribution (94% on average) were classified in the categories of no changes to 1–2 changes. Across all three years, one single item was repeatedly observed as the most frequent negative change: "playing with balloons."

Changes in overall safety scores

The overall household safety scores are presented in Table 6.4. As noted earlier, these are the means of the scores of all items across all households in each visit. At the descriptive level, the second visit scores were higher compared with those of the first visit, across all three years of the program. In order to determine whether these differences are statistically significant, a series of three dependent samples t-tests was conducted. The differences reached statistical significance in the first year ($t(66)=3.16$, $p<.01$), in the second year ($t(68)=8.99$, $p<.005$), and in the third year ($t(22)=4.54$, $p<.005$).

Table 6.4 Mean scores for the first and second visits, for all households

Visit score	First year (N=67)		Second year (N=69)		Third year (N=23)	
	Mean	SD	Mean	SD	Mean	SD
First visit	21.8	2.6	19.9	4.4	20.3	5.3
Second visit	22.8	2.3	23.1	2.9	25.4	5.1

Discussion

The current work examined the effectiveness of the home visits intervention program conducted among Israeli Arab families. Across all three years of the intervention, safety scores of the second visits were significantly higher compared with the first visit. We concluded that the home visits initiative, conducted by using structured checklists and delivered by grandmothers living in the nearby geographic area of the intervention, may be effective in improving overall house safety and in encouraging the acquisition of new safety practices among Israeli Arab families.

This intervention may be described as an active education program including home visits, safety assessments of the overall house environment, and distribution of safety devices. While there is previous evidence in support of such interventions, it remains unresolved which of these components—the visit, the assessment, or the safety device distribution—is directly related to the improvement in safety scores, or whether all of these components have an aggregated effect.[15] Furthermore, conducting randomized controlled trials to assess the effectiveness of "home visits" in the context of Israeli Arab children is needed to provide additional support of the findings reported in this intervention.

Grandmothers as agents of social change constitute a critical and unique part of this innovative program. The engagement of grandmothers represents one aspect of senior citizen engagement in civic life. While the literature on this topic is sparse, researchers have pointed to the important role of senior citizens in assuming functions that the government and private sector have either abandoned or never assumed. In the United States, Jirovec and Hyduk assert that we are "in an era of diminishing governmental responsibility for human services," raising concerns among social welfare professionals, who are "likely to have more involvement with nonprofit, voluntary agencies and more duties related to the development and evaluation of volunteer programs and services."[16] In Britain, the "aging population is being redefined as a social, political and economic opportunity,"[17] with older citizens valued for their contribution to the market economy through paid or unpaid workforce participation. At the same time, the MacArthur studies of "successful aging" and longevity document the positive impact of senior citizen participation in social activities, including civic engagement.[18]

The volunteering grandmothers of this initiative learned many of the practical aspects of community activism. These grandmother activists additionally mapped the dangers children confront as they walk to school. The "grandmas" lobbied the Mayor and other local decision makers to improve infrastructure and achieve the removal of dangerous garbage strewn in the streets. To summarize, although the primary goal of the intervention was to improve child safety, this project also demonstrated the potential social, cultural, and political implications of the child safety intervention program using grandmothers as agents of social change not only in terms of improving child safety but also as a means to incorporate senior citizens as full partners in civic life.

The current work has several limitations. The first is the sampling method, specifically, the absence of randomization and use of a control group. This limits the ability to draw firm conclusions about the effectiveness of the intervention and its direct role in improving safety scores. Additionally, the sample sizes were relatively small. Another limitation concerns the nature of the relationship between the participating mothers and the volunteering grandmother instructors. As noted, the instructors were senior women from the local community. Given that the community examined was characterized by close relationships and a great deal of familiarity, it is likely that the instructors had some previous acquaintance with the participating mothers. Such familiarity may have affected the nature of the home visits and motivation to assimilate the recommended changes. Moreover, we focused on one specific setting—a local Arab community in the Northern District of Israel. Focusing on a specific context, however exploratory by nature, limits the capacity to generalize the findings to different settings and populations.

Findings from the current work raise several important and interesting questions. For example, our initiative did not address the nature of the changes made following the intervention. In fact, the checklist questionnaire can be classified into two major categories of potential changes: "hard changes," that is, changes that involve altering one's physical environment, which may require financial investment (for example, the installation of a fence or other mechanism to separate play and parking areas; installing window bars to limit the opening of windows), versus "soft changes," which may demand altering one's thinking and habits, as well as the investment of time and/or effort, but do not generally entail financial outlay (for example, keeping a close eye on the children while they are eating; prohibition of playing with balloons). A preliminary investigation indicates that the soft changes were made more frequently than the equivalent hard changes. A more systematic examination of this question may shed light on the nature of the changes most inspired by the home visits intervention plan, and whether these tendencies might change between different groups based on their economic status. Another potential avenue for research relates to the longitudinal nature of our findings. While in our intervention the participants received a second home visit several months after the first, future studies should aim for a more extended frame of reference—for example, whether the safety improvements are still evident in the year following the first visit, or if, instead, this type of intervention is limited in its long-term effects.

The results from the current intervention may be utilized by policy makers in their efforts to reduce safety gaps between Jewish and Arab children in Israeli homes. Providers of primary health care services may include home visits in their safety-promotion strategy and train local instructors to administer such education. As recently summarized in the journal *Pediatrics*,[19] it is important that these educational interventions go beyond considering the acquisition of new knowledge to highlight the impact of the intervention on at-risk behaviors. Cultural sensitivity is another key aspect; scholars and practitioners should not overlook the unique needs and capabilities of the specific population discussed in their efforts to increase child safety among low-income populations throughout the world.

Three additional points need to be made about this initiative. First, this chapter has reported on only one fairly small part of the overall child safety HATD initiative with Beterem, one that was best implemented from a scientific point of view. In fact, this four-year intervention worked with hundreds of young mothers—both Palestinian and Jewish—all in Israel. Second, in recognition of the accomplishments of this initiative, Beterem won the 2018 Israeli Minister of Welfare award, and it placed second at the 2017 Safe Kids Worldwide Childhood Injury Prevention Convention (PrevCon).

Finally, from an HATD perspective, we are encouraging the dissemination of this initiative into other communities, such as the ultra-Orthodox Jewish neighborhood of Bnei Brak. Our aim is to bring the Jewish grandmothers together with the Arab grandmothers so that the latter can pass on their lessons learned, measurably decreasing childhood accidents, and at the same time continue the process of "healing across the divides," in this case between Palestinians living in Israel and Israeli Jews. Our hope, again from the HATD perspective, though much more challenging from a political point of view, is to someday implement this initiative in both Israel and the Occupied Palestinian Territory.

Notes

1 Center for Disease Control, (2008) CDC Childhood Injury Report Available at: https://www.cdc.gov/safechild/child_injury_data.html Accessed: June 13, 2020.
2 Ellsasser, G. (2006). Epidemiological analysis of injuries among children under 15 years of age in Germany. The starting point for injury prevention. *Gesundheitswesen, 68* (7), pp: 421–428.
3 Barcelos, R.S., Del-Ponte. B., & Santos, I.S. (2018). Interventions to reduce accidents in childhood: a systematic review. *Jornal de Pediatria*; *94*(4), pp: 351–367. doi: 10.1590/0102-311X00139115.
    Kendrick, D., Barlow, J., Hampshire, A., et al. (2008). Parenting interventions and the prevention of unintentional injuries in childhood: systematic review and meta-analysis. *Child: Care, Health & Development, 34*(5), pp: 682–695.
4 Phelan, K.J., Khoury, J., Xu, Y., et al. (2011). A randomized controlled trial of home injury hazard reduction: the HOME injury study. *Archives of Pediatrics & Adolescent Medicine, 165*(4), pp: 339–345.
    Orton, E., Whitehead, J., Mhizha-Murira, J., et al. (2016). School-based education programs for the prevention of unintentional injuries in children and young people (Review). *Cochrane Database of Systematic Reviews, 12.*
5 Kendrick, D., Ablewhite, J., Achana, F., et al. (2016). *Keeping Children Safe: a multicenter program of research to increase the evidence base for preventing unintentional injuries in the home in the under-fives.* Southampton (UK): NIHR Journals Library; 2017 Jul. (Programme Grants for Applied Research, No. 5.14.) Available from: https://www.ncbi.nlm.nih.gov/books/NBK447053/. Accessed: June 27, 2020.
6 Stewart, T. C., Clark, A., Gilliland, J., et al (2016). Home safe home: Evaluation of a childhood home safety program. *Journal of Trauma Acute Care Surgery,* 81(3), pp: 533–540.
7 Pomerantz, W., Gittleman, M., Hornung, R., et al. (2012). Falls in children birth to 5 years: different mechanisms lead to different injuries. Journal of *Trauma and Acute Care Surgery, 73*(3), pp: 254–257.
8 Campbell, M., Lai, E.T.C., Pearce, A. et al. (2019). Understanding pathways to social inequalities in childhood unintentional injuries: findings from the UK millennium cohort study. *BMC Pediatri*cs, *19*, p. 150.

 9 Birken, C.S., Macarthur. C. (2004). Socioeconomic status and injury risk in children. *Pediatrics & Child Health, 9*(5), pp: 323–325.

10 Baron-Epel, O. & Ivancovsky, M. (2013). A socio-ecological model for unintentional injuries in minorities: a case study of Arab Israeli children. *International Journal of Injury Control and Safety Promotion, 22,* pp: 48–55.

11 Nir, N., Ophir, Y., Weiss, O., et al. *Child injuries in Israel: 'Beterem' National Report 2017.* Petach-Tikva: 'Beterem - Safe Kids Israel', Publication No. 1100, October 2017.

12 Ibid.

13 Martinson, M. & Minkler, M. (2006). Civic engagement and older adults: A critical perspective. *The Gerontologist, 46,* pp: 318–324.

14 Kendrick, D., Barlow, J., Hampshire, A., et al. (2008). Parenting interventions and the prevention of unintentional injuries in childhood: systematic review and meta-analysis. *Child: Care, Health & Development, 34*(5), pp: 682–695

15 Elkan, R., Kendrick, D., Hewitt, M., et al. (2000). The effectiveness of domiciliary home visiting: a systematic review of international studies and a selective review of the British literature. *Health Technology Assessment, 4*(13), pp: 1–339.

16 Jirovec, R. L. & Hyduk, C. A. (1998). Type of volunteer experience and health among older adult volunteers. *Journal of Gerontological Social Work, 30,* pp: 29–42.

17 Biggs, S., (2001). Toward a critical narrativity: Stories of aging in contemporary social policy. *Journal of Aging Studies, 15,* p. 310.

18 Rowe, J. (2011). Successful societal adaptation to the aging of America. *Public Policy & Aging Report, 21*(4), pp: 11–16.

19 Council on Community Pediatrics. (2009). The role of preschool home-visiting programs in improving children's developmental and health outcomes. *Pediatrics, 123* (2), pp: 598–603.

Chapter 7

Family Defense Society

Decreasing obesity and early detection of domestic violence in refugee camps and metropolitan Nablus, Occupied Palestinian Territory

Norbert Goldfield

Introduction

While focusing on one particular grantee, the Family Defense Society (FDS), this chapter highlights the many interventions that Healing Across the Divides has sponsored on aspects of the physical health of women. In the introduction, I will briefly discuss the research in one particular area, obesity in Palestinian women, both in Israel and the Occupied Palestinian Territory (OPT). I will also touch on the challenge of domestic violence against women in the OPT (see chapter 10 for an extended discussion surrounding this critical topic, which is the subject of several HATD-supported interventions). The Family Defense Society (FDS) began its work as the only shelter in the West Bank for Palestinian women fleeing domestic violence. The FDS decided to work on decreasing obesity, in part, as a way to engage with and identify as early as possible women who were at risk for domestic violence.

I will then turn to the approach that the FDS undertook in this HATD-funded initiative, followed by results. In the concluding comments, I will reflect on the role of an American organization such as HATD in tackling health issues such as obesity and, to a certain extent, violence against women in a setting of ongoing conflict such as the Israeli-Palestinian conflict.

While obesity is increasing throughout the world, a noteworthy socioeconomic and geographic component can be observed. The greatest increase is occurring in the Middle East, sub-Saharan Africa, and India.[1] Obesity among Arab populations is growing at an alarming rate.[2] Recent interventions have documented that relatively inexpensive interventions can decrease obesity in Palestinian women.[3] Two interventions, in particular, formed part of the basis for the work that the FDS undertook. These are the Chronic Disease Self-Management Program (CDSMP), developed at Stanford University,[4] and the findings of the recently published study "Lifestyle Intervention in Obese Arab Women," which focused on Arab communities in Israel.[5]

Domestic violence against women, including Palestinian women, is, tragically, an issue affecting women throughout the world. According to a Human Rights Watch report from 2006,

> A significant number of women and girls in the Occupied Palestinian Territories (OPT) are victims of violence perpetrated by family members and intimate partners. While there is increasing recognition of the problem and some Palestinian Authority (PA) officials have indicated their support for a more forceful response, little action has been taken to seriously address these abuses. Indeed, there is some evidence the level of violence is getting worse while the remedies available to victims are being further eroded.[6]

Fast forward to 2019: "A recent report from the United Nations Population Fund found, in a survey, that nearly 1 in 3 Palestinian women suffered from 'psychological, physical, sexual, social or economic violence by their husbands at least once during the preceding 12 months.'"[7]

Background on the FDS

The Family Defense Society (FDS) is a Palestinian women's nonprofit organization founded in 1994 by a group of female professionals based in Nablus in the northern part of the Occupied Palestinian Territory. The FDS aims to improve the status of Palestinian women and children. FDS's mission is to help women in the OPT play a significant role in developing local society. In its efforts to empower and protect Palestinian women in the OPT, the FDS has three main objectives:

- The defense, protection and empowerment of women who face psychological, sexual, and physical abuse;
- Protection for abused girls, women, and their children; and

- Raising awareness within the Palestinian community of violence against women and fostering, in general, women's rights.

Prior to the HATD-funded initiative, the FDS established and continues to operate:

1 The first shelter for Palestinian women and children at immediate physical risk;
2 A legal empowerment program; and
3 A social empowerment program that provides economic and social support services, including vocational training, for women in need. This program also operates a 24/7 help line.

Objectives of the HATD-funded intervention:

1 Highlighting the effects of obesity on women's health, social, and psychological well-being;
2 Defining the best methods for combating the epidemic effects of obesity on women and laying the groundwork for practical initiatives to combat this risk;
3 Taking practical initiatives to raise awareness among women in the community on the risks of obesity and methods for combating it; and
4 Specifying future initiatives based on the findings and outcomes of this pilot project.

Method

This initiative is guided by two evidence-based interventions: the Chronic Disease Self-Management Program (CDSMP) developed at Stanford University and the findings of the recently published study "Lifestyle Intervention in Obese Arab Women," which focused on Arab communities in Israel. The FDS program started in October 2016 and consisted of training the FDS leadership using the CDSMP. On completion of this phase, the FDS continued with a Train the Trainer (ToT) course for eighteen educators in three fields: nutrition, sports, and psychosocial support. The ToT ran for twenty hours. At the same time, FDS and HATD staff reviewed the "Lifestyle

Intervention" article, spoke with the authors of the study, and adapted some of the instruments used for evaluation of that study for use in this intervention.

During the first six months, the 18 FDS trainers reached 192 beneficiaries. During the first year, the FDS worked with a total of 314 women in Nablus Old City and Balata, Askar, and Al-Ain refugee camps. The activities took place in twelve locations in cooperation with local community organizations. The first year ended with an "open day," which took place in Nablus on October 11, 2017. At this gathering, beneficiaries presented project findings to the Palestinian Ministry of Health, Ministry of Social Development, and partner non-governmental organizations (NGOs). The second year replicated and expanded on the activities of the first. In the third year, 500 women from different geographic regions in the governorate were targeted. Pre- and post-intervention questionnaires were distributed. The questionnaire combined physical data such as body mass index (BMI) with an Arabic translation of the Dartmouth COOP charts, a self-completed instrument measuring health status.[8] The following analysis report shows the results of 250 pre- and 250 post-intervention questionnaire forms.

Results

Demographic data

All participants were women: 68% were under 40 years old, 32% older than 45; 60% of participants had four children or more, 40% had three children or fewer or none; 80% were married, 20% single. The following tables demonstrate health behavior changes over time (Tables 7.1–7.5).

Before the program started, more than 60% of women agreed that their prime motivation for losing weight was prompted by how people viewed them. After the program, 78% of the women stated that their motivation behind losing weight was the health dangers of obesity. Interestingly, in the pre-intervention questionnaire, most women believed that exercise should only be done in sports facilities. In contrast, in post-intervention questionnaire forms, women indicated that

Table 7.1 Weight

Weight	Pre	Post
Less than 70kg	26%	38%
70–80	37%	41.2%
80 and more	37%	20.8%

Table 7.2 Body Mass Index (BMI)

BMI	Pre	Post
18.5–25	16%	30%
26–30	30%	38%
31–35	36%	22%
36 and more	18%	10%

Table 7.3 Exercise per week

Exercise	Pre	Post
None	28.2%	6%
Less than 10 minutes	22.6%	8.2%
10-15 minutes	16.6%	12.6%
16-20	6.6%	24.2%
21-30	15.6%	14%
30 minutes and more	10.4%	36%

Table 7.4 Sleep

Sleep amount	Pre	Post
Less than 5 hours	45%	3.6%
5 hours	12.5%	4.0%
6 hours	23.3%	32%
7 and more	19.2%	60.4%

Table 7.5 Average water intake

Water	Pre	Post
Less than 1 liter	27.8%	8.4%
1 liter	32.0%	10.9%
2 liters	24%	42.6%
3 liters and more	16.2%	38.1%

Table 7.6 Food quantities

Daily practice	Pre (Not difficult)	Post (Not difficult)
Do not eat between main meals	72.8%	84.8%
Eat breakfast daily	72.2%	94%
Reduce the amount of sugar and fat	56.6%	80.2%
Prepare meals that do not cause obesity	28%	80%
Physical activity at home	19%	78.2%
Practice walking or running	41.2%	68.9%

exercise could be carried out anywhere. Many stated that one could exercise while doing housework or watching television (such as doing leg exercises, yoga, or tai chi).

The percentage of those who drank less than 1 liter of water per day decreased significantly after the intervention. The consumption of foods that caused obesity decreased as seen in Table 7.6. The percentage of women eating fresh vegetables increased from 46% before the program to 80%. The consumption of fried vegetables decreased to 36% from 90%.

Individual stories

Samah is a woman aged 35 years who completed elementary school, weighed almost 200 pounds, and felt that it was hopeless trying to lose weight. She had tried diet programs before joining the FDS sessions but had failed to lose weight. Even though hesitant at first, she joined the FDS program and attended all the sessions. Initially, she participated in the sessions without engaging or asking questions. After she lost weight, she started speaking about her personal experiences within the group. She volunteered to speak to women about the difficulty any woman faces beginning a program such as the FDS program and the positive feeling she experienced when she became part of the FDS group dynamic. She lost almost 26 and a half pounds (12 kilograms). She changed her lifestyle completely, resulting in renewed mental and physical energy.

The FDS-trained health workers at the Watany Hospital (a government hospital in Nablus) adapted the CDSMP program to engage with and educate patients with chronic diseases while waiting to see the doctor. The health workers used the same techniques taught by FDS to help patients understand how to manage their diseases. The health workers also distributed brochures put out by the FDS. FDS also engaged with the Palestinian Ministry of Health, as the FDS has historically sought ways to engage with governmental institutions focused on health.

Discussion

This initiative by the FDS staff to tackle obesity among Palestinian women has had a significant impact both on participants and the organization. At the participant level, the intervention succeeded not just in reducing obesity but also, among other effects, in bringing about improved sleep patterns and increased exercise, both of which are tied to obesity. At the organizational level, this HATD-funded initiative significantly influenced FDS strategy and operations. Adapting a classification specified in the publication *Promoting Health through Organizational Change*, one can divide HATD's impact into the following categories: strengthening capacities for improvement; identifying strategic directions in behavior change; conducting a critical functions analysis; and improvement using rapid cycle change.[9]

Strengthening capacities for improvement

First, by way of background, while all proposals to HATD must be innovative, our decision making concerning the approval of a grant to a CBO in Israel versus the OPT is different. That is, the implementation of the Stanford CDSMP as part of the strategy of this initiative in the OPT is innovative. We also recognize that Israel has a health system, whereas the OPT has health care organizations that under certain circumstances are responsive to the Palestinian Ministry of Health in either the West Bank or Gaza. Thus, for example, if there is already existing literature on both the scientific validity and the cost-effectiveness of a health care intervention that is not widely disseminated (our definition of "innovative"), we will not fund such an intervention in Israel because it has a health system. There are Israeli national bodies that could decide to fund the CDSMP and, for example, include the CDSMP in the "national basket of services" (a health service covered for all Israelis). We funded the initiative in the OPT as it is both scientifically valid, low cost, and cost-effective. In so doing, we hope that either additional Palestinian organizations (both private and/or the Ministry of Health) will adopt the CDSMP and other aspects of what the FDS has accomplished or that the organization will engage with the FDS to implement the program in other parts of the OPT.

Strengthening community-based organizational capacity goes to the heart of what HATD aims to accomplish in its work. Batalden and Nolan describe four key ingredients for making continuous quality improvement (CQI) an integral part of the organization: "leadership, investment in improvement, professional subject matter knowledge and knowledge for improvement."[10]

Assessing the ability of the leadership of a community-based organization (CBO) to effectively implement an innovative HATD-funded program is a critical first step in HATD's decision-making process in deciding whether or not to fund an initiative. Such an evaluation is very challenging. We base our assessment of leadership on in-person/on-site meetings; a detailed application proposal that includes how the CBO intends to evaluate its efforts; and a group meeting with the leadership of all CBOs applying for a grant.

Both before and, if accepted, after the start of an initiative we ask the following questions/make the following statements pertaining to organizational evaluation and improvement: What outcomes are you looking for as a result of your initiative? What type of information, in general, do you need to achieve these outcomes? We communicate to the CBO leadership: whatever information you want to collect to improve your organization internally as you assess this initiative that HATD has funded is the information that we would like to see and read. Our philosophy is that we are not interested in external evaluations. We encourage internally generated continuous quality improvement (CQI). This is all the information we are interested in. We ask the CBO leadership to share with us the details on process and outcomes measures they wish to track. If they are not evidence-based, then HATD's role is to point this out and make suggestions of evidence-based approaches. If the leadership is strong, the CBO will generally engage with our suggestions and we will come to an agreement satisfactory to both the CBO and HATD.

After we accepted its general proposal, the FDS leadership immediately accepted our suggestions to review the paper published in the *Archives of Internal Medicine* referenced above for lessons that could be adapted for the FDS intervention. This paper documented the impact of an intervention on obesity on Palestinian women living in Israel.

In addition, the FDS leadership enthusiastically participated in and learned the Chronic Disease Self-Management Program (CDSMP), which, with its translation into Arabic, represented an important part of an effective intervention for obesity among Palestinian women. This commitment on the part of the FDS leadership pointed to its strength and the group's "investment in improvement, professional subject matter knowledge and knowledge for improvement."

Identifying strategic directions in behavior change

It is true that "high performing organizations achieve success by identifying and concentrating efforts on a small number of strategic directions." Yet this aspiration is especially challenging for Palestinian organizations in the OPT. These CBOs have very limited access to funds over the long term. HATD is too small to be able to make indefinite commitments or to pledge core funding of specific organizations (though this option has been discussed at the board level). As a consequence, most Palestinian CBOs often have to adjust their strategic direction based on the availability of funds. That said, it is impressive that the FDS applied for a grant with the innovative idea of intertwining an obesity intervention with one of their core programs, the shelter for women at risk for domestic violence.

Thinking about sustainability of the intervention is an ongoing "strategic" direction for any organization in the OPT. As an organization engaged in both funding and provision of organizational consulting, HATD is continuously exploring new opportunities for partnerships and funding opportunities for organizations in the OPT such as the FDS. This is a critical element of HATD's work, especially in the OPT.

Conducting a critical functions analysis

A "critical functions analysis" supports staff and clients in their goal of achieving health behavior change. Critical functions that the FDS tapped into in working on this initiative encompassed professional development (for example, learning about the CDSMP); establishing linkages/networks among services and resources (for instance, working with the Palestinian Ministry of Health and other HATD grantees, such as the Ahli Balatah Al-Balad Club, or ABBC) and developing options for help, including self-help groups such as those organized via the CDSMP.

Improvement using rapid cycle change

This is more of an ideal than a reality, in any organization, whether or not it is funded by HATD. HATD has a mechanism in place for the possible implementation of rapid cycle change. That is, every grantee has to submit reports every six months. These reports include data from the grantee's self-evaluation, together with its action plans detailing what the organization intends to do with its results.

Conclusion

Domestic abuse of women is a scourge throughout the world, including the OPT. The leadership of the FDS, which established the first women's shelter in the West Bank, creatively stepped out of its comfort zone in applying for an HATD grant dealing with decreasing obesity within the community, a significant medical problem among Palestinian women. In implementing this initiative, the FDS not only decreased obesity, it also increased telephone calls and other engagements from women seeking advice and help for domestic abuse. The group has made substantial strides in its own organizational effectiveness, with the result that the FDS leadership, with the tools it has learned, continues to expand its impact on Palestinian society. Its accomplishments owe much to the strength of its considerable efforts. In addition, the FDS gained a great deal of expertise and political acumen through its work with organizations such as ABBC and political entities such as the Palestinian Ministry of Health, connections that were facilitated by HATD.

Notes

1 Wild, S., Roglic, G., Green, A., et al. (2004) Global prevalence of diabetes estimates for the year 2000 and projections for 2030. *Diabetes Care.* 27(5), pp: 1047–1053.
2 Kalter-Leibovici, O., Atamna, A., Lubin, F., et al. (2007) Obesity among Arabs and Jews in Israel: a population-based study. *Isr Med Assoc* J. 9(7), pp: 525–530.

3 Ofra Kalter-Leibovici, MD; Nuha Younis-Zeidan, MSc; Ahmed Atamna, MD et al. (2010) Lifestyle intervention in obese Arab women: a randomized controlled trial. *Arch Intern Med* 170 (11), pp: 970–976.

4 See https://www.selfmanagementresource.com/ for more information.

5 Ofra Kalter-Leibovici, MD; Nuha Younis-Zeidan, MSc; Ahmed Atamna, MD et al. (2010) Lifestyle intervention in obese Arab women: a randomized controlled trial. *Arch Intern Med* 170 (11), pp: 970–976.

6 Human Rights Watch, (2006) A question of security: violence against Palestinian women and girls Human Rights Watch Available at: https://www.hrw.org/reports/2006/opt1106/; Accessed: June 17, 2020.

7 United Nations Office for the Coordination of Humanitarian Affairs, (2019) Almost one in three Palestinian women reported violence by their husbands in 2018–2019. Occupied Palestinian Territory. Available at: https://www.ochaopt.org/content/almost-one-three-palestinian-women-reported-violence-their-husbands-2018–2019. Accessed: June 17, 2020.

8 Jenkinson, C., Mayou, R., Day, A., et al. (2002) Evaluation of the Dartmouth COOP charts in a large-scale community survey in the United Kingdom, *Journal of Public Health*, 24 (2), pp: 106–111.

9 Skinner, H. (2002) *Promoting health through organizational change.* San Francisco: Benjamin Cummings, p. 149.

10 Batalden, P. and Nolan, T. (1993) *Knowledge for the leadership of continual improvement in health care* AUPHA manual of health services management. Rockville, MD: Aspen Publishers.

Chapter 8

Hadassah Optimal

Exercise and nutrition in the immediate postpartum period in Israel—a successful intervention accompanied by government adoption

Chen Stein-Zamir, Gina Verbov, Rani Polak and Naama Constantini

Introduction

After a dozen years of operation, we are excited to have the opportunity to review the Public Health Nurses Promoting Healthy Lifestyles program (PHeeL-PHiNe), which ran in Israel from 2008 to 2017.[1] In order to promote the health of the entire family, this program focused on training public health nurses working in community-based Mother and Child Health Centers (MCHC) in new exercise and healthy eating initiatives for the mothers, fathers, and children they serve. The main partners were the Ministry of Health (MoH), Israel, and Hadassah Optimal, then the center for health and fitness of Hadassah Medical Center, Jerusalem, and the Heidi Rothberg Sports Medicine Center of Shaare Zedek Medical Center, Hebrew University, Jerusalem. The Jewish Federation of Cleveland Israel Health Advancement for Women (ISHA) and Healing Across the Divides (HATD) provided funding and technical advice.

In 2017, the total population of Israel stood at 9.18 million people, with 184,000 live births annually. Of these births, 74% are Jewish and 21% Moslem; the rest include Christians, Druze, Circassians, and other communities. The PHeeL-PHiNe program ran in three Ministry of Health districts in Israel, starting first in the Jerusalem District and later in the Northern and Southern Districts. Of the total number of births in Israel, some 35,000 (19%) were registered in the Jerusalem District, some 22,000 (12%) in the Northern District, and nearly 30,000 (16.3%) in the Southern District.[2] Children aged 0–17 years make up about one-third of the Israeli population.

As described by Rubin et al., in Israel, all children, regardless of age, sex, ethnic group, religion, nationality, or country of origin, are entitled through the National Health Insurance Law to curative and preventive health care services.[3] However, this universal right to health care has not eliminated disparities in health indicators between different populations within the country.

The Ministry of Health (MoH) bears national responsibility for ensuring the health of the population of Israel and strives to achieve this aim by upholding the basic right to health for all.[4] A special division has been set up in the Ministry to deal with health disparities and coordinate and fund special programs, such as an intervention in the Southern District to reduce infant mortality among Bedouin Arabs, the population with the highest infant mortality in Israel.[5] As is happening in other industrialized nations, the Israeli population is facing a worrying rise in the prevalence of obesity and its complications. About one in four children in school grades 7–12 are defined as overweight or obese, with the highest prevalence observed among young people in the Arab population.[6] A national program for the promotion of healthy and active lifestyles was initiated in 2012 across all communities and sectors.[7] PHeeL-PHiNe has played a major part in strengthening the important contribution of public health nurses who provide preventive health services to the national program.

The Public Health Services division of the MoH concentrates on the healthy individual from the perspectives of personal, community, and environmental preventive medicine and health promotion, in line with the WHO definition of health promotion.[8] The Public Health division supplies and supervises public health services throughout the country. In order to reach people effectively, the country is operationally divided into seven districts and thirteen sub-districts. These districts and sub-districts are responsible for public health, regulation, disease prevention, and health promotion. In principle and in compliance with legislation, the district health office acts as a "mini" Ministry of Health and, as such, also furnishes services such as the supervision of pharmacies, dental clinics, geriatric hospitals and senior residences, psychiatry and mental health rehabilitation, and mobility and rehabilitation equipment.

As part of the services provided and supervised by the Public Health division, a national network of MCHCs has been offering preventive health services in Israel since the 1920s. The MCHCs play a critical role in reaching families where they live and advising parents regarding the proper care of their children, childhood immunizations, early childhood development, and early detection of disease and disability. The MCHCs, which include a staff of public health nurses who work together with pediatricians, dietitians, social workers, health promotion specialists, and additional health care professionals, are operated mainly by the Israeli Ministry of Health, with some run by the four Health Funds (Israel's managed care organizations) and two municipalities (Jerusalem and Tel Aviv). The services of the MCHCs are available in each district and sub-district, along with a wide range of other Public Health functions and actions described above. Through these services, the district and sub-districts strive to protect and promote the health of their unique populations, in both environmental and social health as well as personal and individually tailored care. This comprehensive approach facilitates the synergy required to ensure the public's health.

The PHeeL-PHiNe program utilized the existing national infrastructure of MCHCs. It aimed to augment the MCHC role as family health centers to promote the health of the whole family. Within the MCHCs, the program worked with the public health nurses, who form the backbone of the MCHC service. The vast majority of the nurses are female, and most of the babies and children who attend the MCHCs are accompanied by their mothers. The MCHC system has recorded many achievements and has been documented as widely used by all population groups.[9]

The PHeeL-PHiNe Program ran in three large districts, each with a very different demographic makeup. It began with a pilot in the Jerusalem District in 2008 and subsequently continued in this district overall until 2011. It ran from 2011 to 2014 in the Northern District and from 2016 until 2017 in the Southern District. Subsequently, the principles and methodologies utilized in the program have been integrated into routine daily activities of MCHC preventive services.

In Israel, preventive health services for families with young children are available in community- based MCHCs in accordance with the national health insurance law.[10] All children are uniformly eligible for MCHC pediatric care free of charge and regardless of residential status. This standardized and universal care offered by the MCHCs can serve as a model for improving social disparities.[11] As the MCHC services are carried out predominately by public health nurses, it was decided to focus the PHeeL-PHiNe training on these nurses in the Jerusalem District and in the Northern District. In the Southern District, school nurses, employed by the Ministry of Health there, also received training. Two research articles have been published about PHeeL-PHiNe, and some of the information appearing here was taken from these articles.[12]

Not surprisingly, the Public Health nurses already possess a wide knowledge of factors affecting healthy lifestyles, especially for infants. PHeeL-PHiNe was introduced with the aims of promoting further personal and professional empowerment and skill set enhancement, so that these nurses can be more effective in addressing lifestyle modifications with parents and, through them, the entire family. PHeeL-PHiNe provided training for public health nurses in both individual counseling of parent clients and group meetings. In accordance with the experiential methods used, the nurses themselves took part in healthy cooking workshops and physical exercise sessions.

Overall, PHeeL-PHiNe trained 660 public health nurses across the country, working in 270 MCHCs of different sizes located in rural and urban areas and serving populations ranging from extremely low to relatively high socioeconomic status. The program reached the families of almost half the number of babies born each year in Israel. Figure 8.1 shows the flow of information in the Jerusalem District.

In each of the three districts the MCHCs serve all populations—predominantly Jewish, as well as Moslem, Christian, and Druze, and within these populations, all ranges of religious observance. The nurses themselves are also Jewish, Moslem, Christian, and Druze. Training courses were delivered in Hebrew and Arabic and training materials were culturally tailored both by language and by content. Nurses were encouraged to use their own experience and knowledge of cultural differences to shape their counseling and their use of the educational materials. The program was developed and delivered by a multidisciplinary team of professionals from medical, nursing, and allied professions: public health, health promotion, public health nutrition, culinary medicine, sports medicine, lifestyle medicine, exercise physiology, and behavioral psychology. This has also contributed to increased cooperation and appreciation between these disciplines.

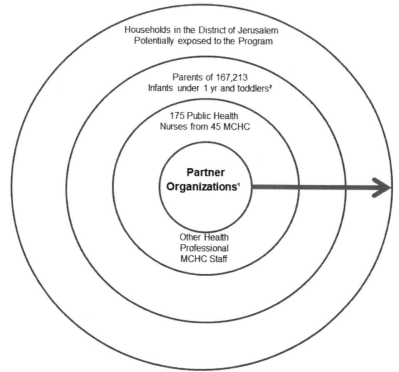

Households in the District of Jerusalem
Potentially exposed to the Program

Parents of 167,213
Infants under 1 yr and toddlers[2]

175 Public Health
Nurses from 45 MCHC

**Partner
Organizations**[1]

Other Health
Professional
MCHC Staff

[1] Center for Lifestyle Medicine, Hadassah University Medical Center
    District Health Office of Jerusalem, Ministry of Health, Israel
    Public Health Department of the Jerusalem Municipality

[2] Average number of infants under 1yr and toddlers attending Jerusalem District
    MCHC 2009-2011. (District Health Office Data Records 2013)

*Figure reproduced from the original that appears in: Polak R, et al Public Health Nurses Promoting Healthy Lifestyles
(PHeeL-PHiNe): methodology and feasibility. *J Ambul Care Manage* (2015) Apr-Jun;38(2):164-77

Figure 8.1 Flow of Information

© *Rani Polak, Naama Constantini, Gina Verbov, et al, The Public Health Nurses Promoting Healthy
Lifestyles (PHeeL-PHiNe): Methodology and Feasibility, Journal of Ambulatory Care Management, 38:2*

On the whole, the program succeeded in registering a marked effect on the health practices of these nurses, particularly in the area of nutrition.[13] In a follow-up study in the Jerusalem District, it was clearly established that nurses who practiced a healthy lifestyle were more likely to provide guidance and counseling to families on healthy behaviors.[14] At baseline, 74% of the nurses reported engaging in any physical activity. This estimate is similar to data found in other studies; for example, Bakhshi found that 75% of registered British nurses in their sample engaged in personal physical activity.[15] At the completion of the PHeeL-PHiNe training course, the number of nurses who engaged in walking (the most frequently reported physical activity) at least once a week had increased by 12%.[16]

Brief literature review

According to the World Health Organization (WHO), a healthy lifestyle is a way of living that lowers the risk of becoming seriously ill or dying early. Not all diseases are preventable, but a large proportion of morbidity and mortality can be avoided by adopting healthy behaviors. However, health is not just about avoiding disease, it is also about physical, mental, and social well-being. A healthy lifestyle is a way of living that can help everyone enjoy more aspects of life.[17]

Ross and Bevans et al. explain that "they (Public Health Nurses) are in a key position to counsel their patients regarding the importance of engaging in healthy lifestyle behaviors such as eating a nutritious diet, participating in regular physical activity, getting adequate sleep, reducing stress, and avoiding tobacco and excessive alcohol intake.... "[18] Studies have shown that as a whole, nurses and student nurses believe that they should have a role in promoting healthy lifestyles and that they should be acting as role models.[19, 20]

In a study of preregistered nurses, Blake et al. concluded that "Educating preregistered nurses about the importance of their own health and well-being and facilitating healthy lifestyle choices at university, on placements, and in their personal lives is an essential but complex task for the future. Improving the health and well-being of preregistered nurses may help to foster positive self-perception and health promotion attitudes that may ultimately have an effect on future patient care. Preregistered nurses should be equipped with early training around core concepts of a healthy lifestyle, including diet, physical activity, and weight management.... "[21]

Perry suggests that if we expect our public health nurses to be the ones to teach our communities about healthy living, then we need to support them as role models. This expectation means exploring ways to ensure that the nurses themselves can eat well and exercise during the day.[22] Promoting healthy lifestyles among nurses has been shown in turn to contribute to successful client interventions.[23] Correspondingly, Owusu-Sekyere also points out that patients are more likely to find health care staff credible if they perceive staff to be following their own healthy lifestyle advice.[24]

Important as it is to provide education and support for nurses to make personal healthy lifestyle choices, it does not always follow that they will feel equipped to counsel others in these areas. For example, about 60% of nurses in a Finnish study found nutrition counseling challenging because of factors such as inadequate knowledge of nutrition.[25] Ljungkrona-Falk et al. described levels of anxiety and uncertainty among nurses, due to lack of knowledge and communication skills, when they were required to discuss children's eating habits with parents.[26]

Experiential learning methods have been used successfully to stimulate deeper understanding in the context of nursing practice. Silberman described experiential learning as the involvement of learners in concrete activities that enable them to experience what they are learning.[27] Murray suggests that experiential learning allows for more engagement by the learner in the learning process.[28] The training stage of PHeeL-PHiNe utilized experiential hands-on learning methods. In this way, not only did the nurses receive knowledge, but they also learned and practiced skills that are relevant in their own personal lives and for their own health. These skills continue to assist them in counseling parents on lifestyle behavior change and the creation of healthier environments for the growth and development of their children.

PHeeL-PHiNe training

Public health nurses participated in all-day weekly training sessions over a period of three months. The format changed slightly in each district, depending on the schedules and availability of the nurses and population characteristics. Participants engaged in both group cooking and group exercise sessions that were aimed at enhancing the nurses' self-efficacy—that is, their confidence in their own ability to carry out these behaviors—and the teaching and encouragement of these behaviors. Course content included interactive lectures and workshops on motivating behavioral change in parents and young children, physical activity, and eating a minimally processed Mediterranean diet, which involved a visit to the supermarket and a session on how to read and understand food labels. Food label literacy is a skill essential to choosing healthier foods. In a Jerusalem study, Sharf et al. established that young adults tended to overestimate their comprehension of food labels. Whereas 44% felt that they understood food labeling very well, only 27% actually received high scores.[29]

Each public health nurse who participated received a personal pedometer, a step-counting device known to motivate individuals to increase their daily walking distance.[30] Since the PHeeL-PHiNe trainings, use of apps on mobile devices to increase physical activity, particularly daily step count, has been increasingly studied. Mobile-phone apps have shown promise in supporting people who have access to smartphones to increase physical exercise.[31]

The first two courses in the Jerusalem District served as a pilot for program development and feasibility and study questionnaire validation. In the Southern District, school nurses also received training, with a course tailored to working with schoolchildren.

Development of educational materials for parents attending the MCHCS

Prior to and during the pilot training of nurses, the different communities served by the MCHCs were researched. This information gathering facilitated the development of culturally and religiously sensitive teaching and educational materials suitable for use with the many and varied MCHC clientele. For example, as part of the pilot in the Jerusalem District, a focus group was carried out with mothers residing in an ultra-Orthodox Jewish community, to understand their families' eating patterns and the effects of religious practices on these patterns. The discussion with community members led to several significant insights that helped to direct the emphases and content of the educational materials produced. As part of the Jewish dietary laws, many ultra-Orthodox families wait for a period of six hours after eating any meat product before eating any milk product. This means that the timing of a midday meat meal affects what can be eaten for an evening meal. The focus group participants, all mothers to several children, described a regular weekday whereby each family member would arrive home at a different time. In practice it was not easy to eat meals together as a family. By the evening, some family members would be able to eat dairy products and some would not. In recognition of this, the importance of plant-based pulses[32] (for example, lentils and chickpeas, which are considered "parev," i.e., neither a meat nor a milk product) was stressed and their nutritional value and versatility in cooking were taught in some detail, including easy recipes. Pulses can also offer an inexpensive yet nutritional option, especially as a source of protein and iron, for communities from all cultures and religions lacking significant financial resources.

The nurses also furnished insights into the cultures and lifestyles of their communities. In order to depict images of people acceptable to all communities, including those conforming to the strictest modesty standards, for the physical activity component, nongender-specific cartoon images were used. Among the materials developed were posters (Figure 8.2 and Figure 8.3), educational games, healthy recipes, table flip charts, and detailed outlines for running workshops with parents. Nurses were encouraged to use the knowledge, skills, and materials acquired during the training in one-on-one sessions with families during scheduled well-baby appointments and in organized group sessions as well as to make any further adaptations of the materials necessary for their communities.

PHeeL-PHiNe programs, 2008–17

PHeeL-PHiNe in the Jerusalem District, 2008–11

The Jerusalem District includes not only the city of Jerusalem but also many outlying towns and municipalities. It covers an area of 627 square kilometers. At that time, the district had 45 MCHCs staffed by 175 public health nurses, serving a multicultural Arab and Jewish population of more than 1,130,000 people annually. Each year, parents of more than 167,000 babies and toddlers received lifestyle counseling, and 640 group meetings for parents outside the individual clinic appointments took place.

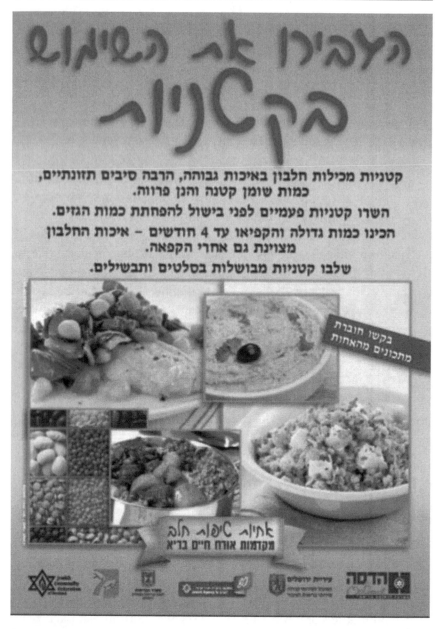

Figure 8.2 Increase your consumption of plant-based pulses

The poster reads:
Pulses contain high-quality protein, a large amount of dietary fiber, a small amount of fat and are parev
(neither a milk product nor a meat product). Soak the pulses twice in water to reduce the amount of gas.
Prepare a large amount and freeze some. It will last for up to four months in the freezer and protein
quality is still excellent after freezing. Combine cooked pulses with salads and other stewed dishes. Ask
the nurse for a recipe booklet!

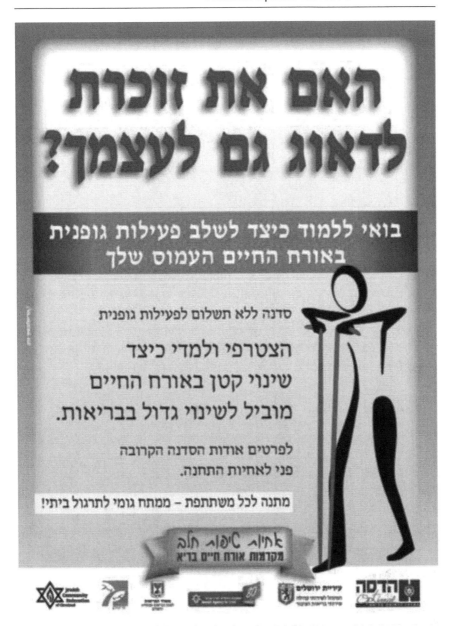

Figure 8.3 Do you remember to also take care of yourself?

The poster reads:
Come and learn how to incorporate exercise into your busy lifestyle. Free exercise workshop. Join us and learn how a small lifestyle change can lead to large health benefits. Ask the nurse for details. A free resistance band for all participants.

PHeeL-PHiNe in the Northern District, 2011–14

With seven times the area of the Jerusalem District, the Northern District at that time had 151 MCHCs staffed by 344 public health nurses, serving a multicultural Arab and Jewish population of more than 1,448,000 people annually. Each year, parents of more than 105,000 babies and toddlers received lifestyle counseling, and 1,380 group meetings for parents outside the individual clinic appointments took place.[33]

PHeeL-PHiNe in the Southern District, 2016–17

The Southern District, the district with the largest area in the country (three times larger than the Northern District), at that time had 48 MCHCs and 141 public health nurses, including 23 public health school nurses, serving a multicultural Arab and Jewish population of more than 1,302,000 people annually. It then had 410 schools attended by the school nurse service provided by the Ministry of Health, covering 15,000 children from grades 1–9. Each year, parents of more than 143,000 babies and toddlers received lifestyle counseling.

Summary of findings

At post-course follow-up, the overall knowledge levels of the nurse participants remained constant, while significant positive changes in attitudes and behaviors were observed when compared with baseline data.[34] Reported weekly exercise increased and dietary habits improved, with a significant increase in the consumption of well-balanced diets. Nurses who practiced healthy lifestyles advised parent clients on healthy behaviors more that those who did not. Nurses with self-reported healthy balanced diets were more than three times more likely to counsel parent clients on healthy cooking and twice as likely to counsel parent clients on physical activity. Follow-up questionnaires filled out 18 months post-course completion in the Jerusalem District showed continued use of course materials and messages in counseling clients and sustained improvements in their personal health behaviors.[35] The pilot intervention stage emphasized the importance of promoting exercise that was practical and financially feasible for the parents, such as walking. Nurses in the pilot trainings reported a tremendous positive experience both from the training course and from the opportunity to run practical group sessions with parents incorporating "hands-on" cooking and physical exercise. The nurses also reported that these sessions strengthened their relationships with parents. This is especially important given that many of the MCHC nurses care for all the children in a family as they are born and throughout the first few years of preschool and school, thus forging a long-term connection with these families. Parents who participated in these sessions appreciated that the information and skills that they received were practical and clear and not complicated "medical speak."

In the Northern District, a "Healthy Lifestyle" component was added to the computerized medical record that the public health nurse completes for every child and parent. During routine appointments, nurses indicate whether the parent has filled out a lifestyle questionnaire and received lifestyle counseling. This feature has helped to ensure the program's sustainability, as the nurses routinely use the accumulated knowledge and skills provided by PHeeL-PHiNe.[36] In the Southern District, 63% of the school nurses who took part in the PHeeL-PHiNe training initiated healthy lifestyle activities in schools, often partnering with teachers and pupils to do so.[37] However, there were indications that the program was not as effective within the Bedouin population in the Southern District.[38] Further investigation of the reasons for this shortfall and for appropriate adaptations of future programs is needed.

PHeeL-PHiNe and beyond

In 2006 the Israeli government launched the national initiative called "Toward a Healthy Future 2020." A major element of this initiative was the national program "You Can Be Healthy" (in Hebrew, "Efsharibari") for the promotion of healthy and active lifestyles for all ages. The program, begun in 2011 and coordinated by the Ministry of Health, partnered with the Ministry of Education and the Ministry of Culture and Sport.[39, 40] The national program for the promotion of healthy and active lifestyles started by focusing on the areas of healthy nutrition and exercise. The PHeeL-PHiNe program has assisted in training public health nurses to play an important part in realizing the aims of this national program. Since the PHeeL-PHiNe trainings took place, the government has recognized that municipalities and regional authorities play an essential role in creating a supportive physical and social environment that can enable families with young children to live a healthy and active life. A citywide element has been added to the national program, partnering with the existing "Healthy Cities" network project and working on furnishing a supportive and enabling environment for the healthy behaviors "prescribed" and encouraged by the MCHC nurses. Joint efforts are crucial for the realization of several of the international Sustainable Development Goals adopted by all United Nations member states in 2015.[41]

More recently, aspects added to the national program for the promotion of healthy and active lifestyles reflect updated policies. A clear policy for a supportive environment for breast-feeding has been endorsed, with training of public health nurses as qualified professional breast-feeding advisers specifically recommended. Another addition is the formation of a national committee on healthy nutrition, which has promoted legislation for a new brightly colored "traffic light" system of nutritional labeling to give consumers a clearer understanding of food products. MCHC nurses also have an important role to play in educating and supporting families with young children in these areas, and PHeeL-PHiNe has helped to equip them with many of the skills to do so.

In conclusion, PHeeL-PHiNe has been shown to be instrumental in increasing the capacity of public health nurses to influence health behaviors of families with babies and young children who attend MCHCs. Moreover, it has assisted nurses in improving and maintaining their own health behaviors, an achievement that helps both the nurses and the families that they counsel. Together with the myriad of other public health services provided by the district and sub-district health offices of Israel, the MCHCs continue to offer a pivotal and quality service for the health of all in Israel.

Notes

1   We would like to thank the District Health Officers, Chief Nurse Supervisors, Public Health Nurses, and staff of the Jerusalem, Northern, and Southern District Health Offices and the Jerusalem Municipality for their active participation, collaboration, and assistance. Thank you to Roni Hasson, Dr. Aliza Stark, and Dana Nir for their invaluable work analyzing the effectiveness of PHeeL-PHiNe.

2 Central Bureau of Statistics Israel, Live Births, Deaths and Infant Deaths by District and Sub-District, Population Group and Religion (2019). https://www.cbs.gov.il/he/publications/DocLib/2019/2.ShnatonPopulation/st02_39x.pdf.

3 Rubin, L., Belmaker, I., Somekh, E., Urkin, J., et al. (2017) Maternal and child health in Israel: building lives *Lancet (2017) 389:10088,* pp: 2514–2530.

4 Ministry of Health Israel, website Available at: https://www.health.gov.il/English/About/Pages/default.aspx Accessed: January 29, 2020.

5 Rubin, L., Belmaker, I., Somekh, E., et al. (2017) Maternal and child health in Israel: building lives *Lancet (2017) 389:10088,* pp: 2514–2530.

6 Ibid.

7 Ministry of Health, Israel "Efsharibari" National Health Promotion Program website Available at: https://www.efsharibari.gov.il/ Accessed: January 29, 2020.

8 World Health Organization (1986, 2005) The Ottawa and Bangkok Charters for Health Promotion. Available at: https://www.who.int/healthpromotion/conferences/6gchp/bangkok_charter/en/. Accessed: January 29, 2020.

9 Zimmerman, D.R., Verbov, G., Edelstein, N., et al. (2019) Preventive health services for young children in Israel: historical development and current challenges *Israel Journal of Health Policy Research* 8 (1), p. 23.

10 Ibid.

11 Shadmi, E. (2018) Healthcare disparities amongst vulnerable populations of Arabs and Jews in Israel. *Israel Journal Health Policy Research* 7(1), p. 26.

12 Polak, R., Constantini, N.W., Verbov, G., et al (2015) Public health nurses promoting healthy lifestyles (PHeeL-PHiNe): methodology and feasibility. *J Ambul Care Manage.* Apr-Jun; 38(2), pp: 164–177.
   Hasson, R., Stark, A.H., Constantini, N., et al. (2018) "Practice what you teach" public health nurses promoting healthy lifestyles (PHeeL-PHiNe): program evaluation. *J Ambul Care Manage.* Jul/Sep; 41(3), pp: 171–180.

13 Ibid.

14 Ibid.

15 Bakhshi, S., Sun, F., Murrells, T., et al. (2015) Nurses' health behaviours and physical activity-related health-promotion practices *British Journal of Community Nursing* (2015) 20 (6), pp: 289–296.

16 Hasson, R., Stark, A.H., Constantini, N., et al (2018) "Practice what you teach" public health nurses promoting healthy lifestyles (PHeeL-PHiNe): program evaluation. *J Ambul Care Manage.* Jul/Sep; 41(3), pp: 171–180.

17 World Health Organization (1999) Healthy living - what is a healthy lifestyle? Available at: https://apps.who.int/iris/handle/10665/108180. Accessed: June 27, 2020.

18 Ross, A., Bevans, M., Brooks, A., et al. (2017) Nurses and health-promoting behaviors: Knowledge may not translate into self-care. *AORN Journal* (2017) 105 (3), pp: 267–275.

19 Darch, J., Baillie, L., Gillison F. (2017) Nurses as role models in health promotion: A concept analysis. *British Journal of Nursing* 26(17), pp: 982–988.

20 Keele, (2019) To role model or not? Nurses' challenges in promoting a healthy lifestyle *Workplace Health & Safety* 67(12), pp: 584–591.

21 Blake, H., Stanulewicz, N., Griffiths, K. (2017) Healthy lifestyle behaviors and health promotion attitudes in preregistered nurses: A questionnaire study. *The Journal of Nursing Education* 56(2), pp: 94–103.

22 Perry, L., (2016) Nurses and midwives need health promotion as much as their patients *International Journal of Nursing Practice* 22 (3), p. 216.

23 Shai, I., Erlich, D., Cohen, A.D., et al (2012), The effect of personal lifestyle intervention among health care providers on their patients and clinics; the promoting health by self experience (PHASE) randomized controlled intervention trial. *Preventive Medicine,* 55(4), pp: 285–291.

24 Owusu-Sekyere, F. (2020) Assessing the effect of physical activity and exercise on nurses' well-being *Nursing Standard.* Available at: https://journals. rcni.com/nursing-standard/evidence-and-practice/assessing-the-effect-of-physical-activity-and-exercise-on-nurses-wellbeing-ns.2020.e11533/pdf. Accessed: June 27, 2020.

25 Ilmonen, J., Isolauri, E., Laitinen, K. (2012) Nutrition education and counselling practices in mother and child health clinics: study amongst nurses. *Journal of Clinical Nursing* 21 (19-20), pp: 2985–2994.

26 Ljungkrona-Falk, L., Brekke, H., Nyholm, M. (2013) Swedish nurses encounter barriers when promoting healthy habits in children *Health Promotion International,* 29(4), pp: 730–738.

27 Murray, R. (2018) An overview of experiential learning in nursing education *Advances in Social Sciences Research Journal 5(1).*

28 Sharf, M., Sela, R., Zentner, G., et al (2012) Figuring out food labels. Young adults' understanding of nutritional information presented on food labels is inadequate. *Appetite* 58(2), pp: 531–534.

29 Sharf, M., Sela, R., Zentner, G., et al (2012) Figuring out food labels. Young adults' understanding of nutritional information presented on food labels is inadequate. *Appetite* 58(2), pp: 531–534.

30 Bravata, D.M., Smith–Spangler, C., Sundaram, V., et al (2007) Using pedometers to increase physical activity and improve health: a systematic review. *JAMA* 298 (19), pp: 2296–3204.

31 Silva, A.G., Simões, P., Queirós, A., et al, (2020) Effectiveness of mobile applications running on smartphones to promote physical activity: A systematic review with meta-analysis *International Journal of Environmental Research and Public Health* 7, p. 2251.

32 Pulses are the edible seeds of plants in the legume family. Pulses grow in pods and come in a variety of shapes, sizes and colors. Available at: https://pulses. org/what-are-pulses#:~:text=Pulses%20are%20the%20edible%20seeds%20 of%20plants%20in,in%20a%20variety%20of%20shapes%2C%20sizes%20 and%20colors. Accessed: June 28, 2020.

33 PHeeL-PHiNe Summary Report prepared for the Jewish Federation of Cleveland and HATD (2014) by Hadassah Optimal.

34 Polak, R., Constantini, N.W., Verbov, G., et al (2015) Public health nurses promoting healthy lifestyles (PHeeL-PHiNe): Methodology and feasibility. *J Ambul Care Manage.* Apr-Jun; 38(2), pp: 164–177.

35 Hasson, R., Stark, A.H., Constantini, N., et al (2018) "Practice what you teach" public health nurses promoting healthy lifestyles (PHeeL-PHiNe): Program evaluation. *J Ambul Care Manage.* Jul/Sep; 41(3), pp: 171–180.

36 PHeeL-PHiNe Summary Report prepared for the Jewish Federation of Cleveland and HATD (2014) by Hadassah Optimal.

37 Nir D, Evaluation of the PHeeL-PHiNe Program in the Israel Ministry of Health Southern District. Undergraduate Thesis. Unpublished (Hebrew) 2018. Faculty of Agriculture Hebrew University of Jerusalem.

38 Ibid.

39 Ministry of Health, Israel "Efsharibari" National Health Promotion Program website. Available at: https://www.efsharibari.gov.il/. Accessed: January 29, 2020.

40 Rosenberg, E., Grotto, I., Dweck, T., et al. (2014) Healthy Israel 2020: Israel's blueprint for health promotion and disease prevention. *Public Health Reviews*. 35. Available at: https://link.springer.com/content/pdf/10.1007%2FBF03391690.pdf. Accessed: June 28, 2020.

41 Marmot, M., Bell, R. (2018) The sustainable development goals and health equity *Epidemiology* 29 (1).

Chapter 9

Kayan

Sustainable new leadership and health improvement for Palestinian women in Northern Israel

Zoe Katzen, Anwar Monsoor, Mona Mahjna, Rafa Anabtawi and Norbert Goldfield

Introduction

Background and setting

Although Palestinians living in Israel have a standard of health characterized as the "highest in the Arab and Muslim world," it is significantly lower than that of Israeli Jews.[1] The life expectancy of Palestinian women is 80 years, compared with 84 for Israeli Jewish women. Mammography rates are lower among Palestinian women living in Israel than those for Israeli Jewish women.[2] Na'amnih and colleagues identified a recent major challenge: the life expectancy gap between Palestinians living in Israel and Jewish Israelis, which narrowed between 1975 and 1998, began widening again in subsequent years.[3] Importantly, the percentage of smokers among Arab Israelis is higher than among Jews, at all age levels. An Israeli Ministry of Health (MoH) report from 2015 states that the share of smokers among Palestinian Arab men living in Israel is twice that of Jewish men: 44% versus 22%, respectively.[4] In contrast, the portion of Palestinian women living in Israel who smoke is much lower than that of Jewish women: 7% versus 15%, respectively. The rate of diabetes is much higher among all Palestinians living in Israel than that of Israeli Jewish women (prevalence of 12% versus 21%).[5] Recent findings document that the Israeli government allocates fewer funds to Palestinian localities in Israel and that Palestinians in Israel are offered fewer economic opportunities than Jews.[6]

Three managed care organizations, a relatively small number of large hospitals, and five medical schools dominate the health care landscape in Israel. In 1995, a new health law was passed that significantly increased coverage to include all Israeli citizens, including Palestinians living in Israel.[7] Access, however, can be a significant challenge.[8] Not only are there relatively fewer inpatient hospital services available for the Arab Israeli population but also, given the average distance of medical facilities from Arab Israeli localities, medical centers are considerably less accessible. The state of Israel established local health committees (LHCs) in the 1990s in an effort to encourage local input into aspects of health care, but these committees have no legal power to make changes in the Israeli healthcare system.

Kayan, a Palestinian feminist organization based in Northern Israel, strives to defend and promote the rights of women and to ensure their integration in decision-making positions. The organization's goal is to eliminate gender disparity among Arab women in Israel. Support of women-led community organizing in Arab villages has emerged as a cornerstone of Kayan's work. Grassroots community activism is integral to Kayan's vision of social change, empowering women to overcome discrimination and improving their lives in tangible ways. At the core of their strategy is the Jusur ("bridges" in Arabic) Forum of Arab Women Leaders, which consists of about 35 women community leaders from approximately twenty villages where Kayan operates. This aspect of Kayan provides a crucial framework for its empowerment work and underpins the sustainability of community-based initiatives for social change.

The initiative

Kayan submitted a proposal to HATD in 2013 to develop sustainable female leadership at a local level in Israel's Northern District. This was accomplished with funding and technical assistance from HATD together with major financial support from the Jewish Federation of Cleveland. Kayan began its effort in three villages and over the next few years expanded the empowerment intervention to five villages while involving Kayan's Jusur Forum of Arab Women Leaders. The model consisted of the following steps:

a   Kayan staff based in Haifa, Israel (the largest city in the Northern District), went to several villages and identified several possible female leaders in these villages.

b   The women that Kayan recruited in each village performed a needs assessment of which health issues they wished to focus on and what they aimed to accomplish.

c   The women then chose the vehicles for addressing the needs that they identified, including one-time lectures on health topics (such as breast cancer), courses (on diabetes, obesity, among others), and participation in local health committees (one of which, for example, sought to have a village implement a walking path).

d   The women in each village decided what to tackle, taking into account their interests, a project's overall feasibility, and the response of local political leadership.

The impact was measured by:

a   Selection and training of agents of social change.
b   Change in knowledge for the agents of social change, participants in village programs, and other political actors in the community.
c   Change in outcomes, particularly changes at the local village level involving the participation of local health committees.

Change in knowledge was measured using questionnaires based on validated questionnaires adapted to the local cultural context.

Results

Kayan implemented this five-year program in Deir Hanna, Jdaydi il Maker, Majd el Krum, Salem, and Yafit el Nasr.

A case report illustrates the extent of change possible at the individual level:

E is a single woman, 40 years old, from Deir Hanna who was referred to the Kayan-sponsored group by the Israeli Welfare Department. She was so introverted that the director of the sports department at the local council, in one of the meetings, mentioned that he lived in her neighborhood but never knew of her existence until the previous year. At the beginning of the empowerment process, E remained silent and found it very difficult to participate in the community activities organized by the group because of the limitations set by her parents. With time, however,

E gradually started to take part in the various group and community activities, and she also began to take a role in organizing the events. As her strengths emerged, the leaders discovered that she proved effective at recruiting new women to activities and demonstrated excellent organizing skills. During the year, she took it upon herself to organize a lecture on her own, resulting in a good-quality lecture and sizable audience attendance. She worked independently during the entire process of organizing the lecture. More recently, E began cooperating with the group members and to carry out activities jointly. E was unemployed, but devoted much of her time to cooking and baking, a hobby she loved. Through the encouragement of the group members, she began making pastries and selling them, and her production soon doubled. In addition, she insisted, over the initial refusal of some members, that her family accept the fiancé she chose. Later on, she decided to leave her fiancé, which was also initially met with rejection by some members of her family. She recruited the support of the Sheikh (community elder or leader), and he assisted her in convincing her parents that this was the right decision for her.

Change also occurred at the village level. For example, a common topic of concern to women in the project was getting exercise, as in many villages there are no usable exercise facilities, and the available spaces (such as community centers, or even public spaces such as parks or streets for running and walking) are intimidating for women to enter, especially since public exercise is still taboo for traditional women of the Palestinian community living in Israel. Creating open spaces where women could exercise required both empowerment for women to claim public spaces or exercise facilities and the framework that would attract women. Thus, in the context of the project, women from the group held public exercise days for women and their families, worked with their community centers to devise inexpensive exercise classes that appealed specifically to women, and made a public outreach effort to bring women to the events offered. The impact of this project has encouraged villages to maintain their exercise programs. The women's group in Arrabeh continues to lead a biweekly walking group, and in 2017 it organized the first-ever women-led marathon, which took place in the heart of the city. The event was in direct response to an incident in which a Palestinian woman was threatened with violence after declaring her intention to run in a public marathon. Thus, it represented a movement not only for women's health but also for women's rights to self-expression and participation in the public sphere as equals.

Approximately 10,000 women participated in individual lectures, courses, local conferences and a national conference that Kayan organized, and direct action or advocacy. Kayan fielded pre- and post-program questionnaires to thousands of women who took some of the health courses (such as those dealing with nutrition, osteoporosis, breast health/cancer) or attended a lecture (such as on appropriate use of medications, diabetes). In one instance, 30 women from the village of Yafit el Nasr participated in a phone questionnaire after attending a series of lectures on nutrition. The questionnaire measured change in knowledge and perceived ability to affect change as a consequence of the interventions. Highlights of the findings included, increases in both knowledge and, to a lesser extent, confidence. Kayan used these results, for each lecture or course, as guideposts for adjustments in its local interventions.

Discussion

This chapter documents the opportunities and challenges of a bottom-up approach to health improvement for one marginalized community: Palestinian women living in Israel. Kayan faced significant hurdles in the implementation of its five-year effort. While Kayan was a pioneer in launching many of the local health committees (LHCs), sustaining them remained a problem throughout the initiative, especially given turnover in representatives following local elections. Not surprisingly, every local women's group requires ongoing support, accompaniment, and resources from Kayan staff to ensure continuity and sustainability. Kayan staff and the local women's groups had very limited help from community activism, in light of the few local NGOs and local health care institutions available for cooperative action and partnerships. Notwithstanding these obstacles, Kayan, together with the five local women's groups it helped create, achieved significant gains. The HATD staff provided not only funding but also technical expertise to measure these gains.

Despite the difficulties of securing ongoing funding for the preservation and growth of these accomplishments, Kayan and these local groups aim to continue and expand on their efforts in a variety of ways. Kayan's staff is committed to attempting to integrate health as a basic human right in all its initiatives. Kayan's leadership views access to health-based knowledge and services not just as a core right for women but as a newfound tool critical to community organizing success. To give one instance, exercise in public without harassment is very much related to the right of women to participate in the public sphere as equals.

Conclusion

Female Palestinians living in Israel have significantly worse health than female Israeli Jews. This initiative to improve their health through developing female leadership was a bottom-up approach, led by local women and facilitated by Kayan, a Palestinian feminist non-health care organization based in Northern Israel. Approximately 10,000 women from five villages (Deir Hanna, Jdaydi il Maker, Majd el Krum, Salem, and Yafit el Nasr) participated.

Kayan, together with the five local women's groups, helped create and achieve significant gains. However, ongoing funding for these bottom-up efforts remains an issue.

Improving health care for marginalized communities constitutes a significant challenge throughout the world. This effort highlights both the obstacles to and accomplishments of health improvement for Palestinian women living in Israel, an area of the world that continues to shed blood. We hope that the success of these local Palestinian women can eventually lead these leaders to have an impact beyond their own communities and even beyond health care.

Notes

1 Chernichovsky, D., Bisharat, B., et al (2017) *The Health of the Arab Israeli Population*. Taub Center for Social Policy Studies in Israel. Jerusalem. https://arabstates.unwomen.org/en/what-we-do/ending-violence-against-women/facts-and-figures#:~:text=Facts%20and%20Figures%3A%20Ending%20Violence%20against%20Women%20and,experienced%20some%20form%20of%20violence%20in%20their%20lifetime. Accessed: October 3, 2018.

2 Hayek, S., Enav, T., Shohat, T., et al. (2017) Factors associated with breast cancer screening in a country with national health insurance: Did we

succeed in reducing healthcare disparities? *Journal of Womens Health* (Larchmt). Feb 2017; 26(2), pp: 159–168.

3 Na'amnih, W., Muhsen, K., Tarabeia, J., et al (2010) Trends in the gap in life expectancy between Arabs and Jews in Israel between 1975 and 2004. *International Journal of Epidemiology*, 39 (5), 1 pp: 1324–1332.

4 Ministry of Health (2016), Minister of Health Report on Smoking in Israel. As quoted in. Chernichovsky et al. op cit.

5 Kalter-Leibovici, O., Chetrit, A., Lubin, F., et al (2012) Adult-onset diabetes among Arabs and Jews in Israel: A population-based study. *Diabetic Medicine* 29(6), pp: 748–754.

6 Lewin, A.C., Stier, H., Caspi-Dror, D. (2006) The place of opportunity: Community and individual determinants of poverty among Jews and Arabs in Israel, *Research in Social Stratification and Mobility* 24 (2), pp: 177–191.

7 Waltzberg, R. and Rosen, B. (2020) *The Israeli Health Care System.* Commonwealth Fund. Available at: https://www.commonwealthfund.org/international-health-policy-center/countries/israel. Accessed: June 17, 2020.

8 Clarfield, A.M., Manor, O., Nun, GB., et al. (2017) Health and health care in Israel: An introduction. *Lancet* 389, pp: 2503–2513.

Chapter 10

Ma'an

Impacting domestic violence against Bedouin women in Southern Israel

Norbert Goldfield and Safa Shehada

Introduction

This chapter will focus on domestic violence, one of the most press-ing problems confronting women and girls throughout the world. The introduction will briefly provide background on the domestic abuse challenge both throughout the world and in Israel in particu-lar. In the remainder of the chapter, we will describe the community organization, Ma'an, that successfully implemented an initiative in this arena, together with the results of this initiative. Of importance, after completion of three years of funding, Ma'an has been able to continue its important work with other sources of funding. We will then analyze HATD's role other than funding, both during the initi-ative and in its continuation.

Domestic violence is a worldwide phenomenon. Statistically, pov-erty, alcohol consumption, low female empowerment (or an unequal position between men and women) are all predictors of domestic vio-lence.[1] It is estimated that 37% of women in Arab countries have expe-rienced domestic violence.[2] According to a United Nations report, approximately 200,000 women were victims of domestic violence in Israel between 2014 and 2015.[3] Most recently, the Association of Relief Centers for Victims of Sexual Assault (ARCVSA) in Israel revealed a substantial spike of 41% in domestic abuse reports in 2018, affecting a total of approximately 51,000 women and girls. Of the sexual assaults reported, 88% were carried out by people the victims knew before-hand.[4] Another survey reported that 40% of Israeli women aged 16 through 48 suffered partner violence.[5]

Recent research by Daoud et al. has documented statistically signif-icant differences in the prevalence of intimate partner violence (IPV) between Arab and Jewish immigrant and nonimmigrant women (67%, 30%, and 27%, respectively) in Israel.[6] Types (physical, verbal, and social) and recurrence of IPV were significantly higher among Arab women. In this analysis, compared with IPV among Jewish nonimmigrants, IPV among Arab women persisted after considering socioeconomic, sociodemographic, and reproductive factors. Low family income was the main risk factor for IPV for all women. Among Arab women, IPV was associated with younger age, high religiosity, and living in urban settings.

Turning to the ethnic minority that Ma'an concentrated on in this initiative, the Bedouin population belongs to an indigenous minority, suffering from significant discrimination by the state of Israel. Bedouin women and girls (12 years old and older) number approximately 65,000 in the Negev (Southern Israel) today. This population is exposed to devastating amounts of sexual and gender-based violence (SGBV), including polygamy and domestic violence. Because their freedom and other basic rights are restricted, they are largely unaware of their rights regarding health issues. Notwithstanding the modest efforts carried out by organizations such as Ma'an, awareness of sexual abuse has long been low to nonexistent in the region, and abused women and girls lack knowledge and tools to protect themselves from the abuser. In a setting of SGBV, children are also vulnerable. As psychological and/or physical violence is seen in most Bedouin families as a legitimate way to "discipline" women, this attitude inevitably extends to children in the community, who currently number 110,000 in the Negev (from 0 to 18 years old).

Ma'an

As a grassroots Arab organization based and founded in Beersheva in 2001 and led by Arab female activists, Ma'an is rooted in the community that it serves. It works with the women from the Arab Bedouin community living in the Naqab (Arabic for "Negev"), aiming to improve their lives so they can participate in and contribute to society as equal citizens. Ma'an offers Bedouin women needed advocacy services and emotional support, including a crisis hotline. It is available for free to Bedouin women in the Naqab who urgently need help regarding issues of physical, sexual, and psychological abuse.

The vast majority of the women who call Ma'an's crisis hotline have suffered domestic violence. Bedouin women are facing increasing challenges as a doubly discriminated against minority: because they belong to an ethnic minority and because they are women living in a traditional patriarchal society rife with gender oppression. Bedouin women are economically dependent on their fathers, husbands, or sons. Their access to the public sphere is limited, as is access to educational and employment opportunities. The practice of polygamy further exacerbates the vulnerability of Bedouin women. While it is illegal by Israeli law, approximately 40% of Bedouin families are polygamous. Thus, this phenomenon remains a very significant part of Bedouin women's lives. Given an unemployment rate of approximately 90% for Bedouin women, paying for legal aid is not a realistic option. In addition, women are typically not allowed to leave their villages without a male escort. This makes it even harder for women to get, for example, legal aid (which is unavailable in the villages). These women are unable to turn elsewhere for legal advice and support because of their financial situation and the background of their conservative culture. This description of the challenges confronting Bedouin women provides a backdrop to the Ma'an initiative.

The Ma'an initiative against gender-based violence

Objective of the initiative

Between 2016 and 2019, Ma'an worked to reduce gender-based violence (GBV) in Bedouin society by increasing women's access to support, such as health care and legal services, including the crisis hotline, and by professional engagement to ensure the sustainability of greater support services from the professional community. The following describes what occurred in the three years of the HATD grant.

Year 1 accomplishments

Typically, in year 1 of any HATD grant, the community-based organization (CBO) attempts to document success (or learn from failures) in pilot initiatives. Ma'an in its first year delivered courses to volunteers, who, in turn, provided support to women via a crisis hotline dealing with, in particular, violence and sexual harassment, along with any other health issues. It was designed for Bedouin youth and adults. The 10 volunteers trained in the first year were able to support more than 100 women in the first year. In addition, courses were delivered to community-based professionals working in the field of violence prevention and protection of females. At the same time, Ma'an formed a network of professionals to work on long-term improvements in health and services available for Bedouin women.

In the first year, 124 women called the crisis hotline for the following reasons (Table 10.1):

- 5 women were referred to Ma'an by the police. The women did not want to go to the welfare office as they did not trust it.
- 6 women were referred to a shelter.
- 9 cases were followed up to obtain protection orders from the police and court.

Year 2 accomplishments

In the second year of the project, from December 2016 through November 2017, Ma'an continued with the crisis hotline and set in motion a community health improvement process by creating and supporting local Bedouin women-led networks in targeted villages. HATD suggested the development of this regional network to Ma'an, and it was enthusiastically adopted, although Ma'an staff cautioned that such an effort would not be easy. The objective was to increase Bedouin women's capacity to act as agents of change in improving

Table 10.1 Reasons women call the hotline

Category	Number of calls
Physical Violence	28
Sexual Violence	13
Sexual Harassment	17
Physiological violence	6
Economic violence	24
Threatening	10
Child custody	7
Residency	19
Total	124

community health and, specifically, to fight against SGBV. This was done together with other local partners called local women's committees. During this period, workshops for six groups of women in six locations were conducted as well.

The leadership program, however, faced delays in implementation. To begin with, the search for potential leaders proved challenging. Once they were identified, securing transportation and means of communication for these women posed difficulties, as all come from unrecognized villages (which means they lacked public transportation or any services such as electricity). The villages themselves, such as Zarnouq, are small in population and dispersed over a wide geographic area.

Despite the delays, Ma'an succeeded in establishing leadership groups in six villages, as planned. Ma'an then formed a regional network in which representatives from the six villages met and worked together. Examples of the workshops that Ma'an conducted included:

- Women's rights in national social security such as unemployment benefits and income support
- Personal skills training
- Women's rights at work
- Awareness-raising workshop organized by "One in Nine," a prior HATD grantee, on breast cancer
- "Me and you will change the world": Workshop on the role of leaders
- Screening of the movie *Wajda*, followed by a discussion about women's rights
- Awareness-raising workshop about types of violence against women
- Awareness-raising workshop on nutrition
- Violence against women and its repercussions

After group cohesion was established, local women's committees were formed in each of the localities in cooperation with the municipality, religious leaders, NGO representatives, and female activists. Another committee assessed the needs in each locality and decided on interventions with participating communities. The members of the committee that assessed the needs in each locality also discussed future cooperation and activities for the project.

Beyond these core objectives, other outcomes were achieved. Several of the leaders signed up to work on the crisis hotline. In part as a consequence of the joint meetings between HATD grantees that HATD continues to sponsor regularly, Ma'an and the women's committees established working relations with a number of other groups, including Beterem and One in Nine. In fact, these relationships strengthened to the point that One in Nine presented at some of the workshops that Ma'an organized in its leadership development program. The new regional leadership effort also successfully built relationships with local community councils and managed care organizations (Kupat Holim).

Year 3 accomplishments

In the third and last year of HATD funding, Ma'an kept the crisis hotline going, and the women's committees led groups in the six villages. However, Ma'an's main achievement in this third year was the development and implementation of the "16 Days of Activism Campaign against GBV." The regional network of Bedouin women leaders that Ma'an created implemented that campaign. The regional network leaders produced posters and announcements for television and radio. The posters made their way into demonstrations held, sadly, often around the murder of a woman. Significantly, for many Bedouin women, attendance at these demonstrations was the first time they "came out of the closet" and stood up for their rights. Just as important, men also joined the protests.

As part of the campaign, the women of the regional network and Ma'an decided to publish a video as an awareness raiser on GBV as well as a manifestation of their efforts and skills to conduct campaigns. The video, titled *Discussion behind Masks*,[7] featured 12 women, each of whom wore a mask. They delivered 12 messages representing the 12 months of the year, as an indicator that such campaigns and work are sustainable and should be active all year long. The video led to discussions on social media on violence against women, motivating 9 women to approach Ma'an asking to be members of the network and participate in activities. Judging from "shares" of participants, the video reached approximately 14,000 people on Facebook and another

4,000 on WhatsApp (the video can be found via the link https://bit. ly/2KOpKzn). The campaign was followed by increased interaction with Ma'an's Facebook page and WhatsApp.

This campaign differed from any other campaign that Ma'an had ever undertaken in being based on the collective efforts of women in the regional network. Each and every woman added a post of the day to her WhatsApp story. Women outside the network also contributed postings, which the campaign appended. Sadly, the women of the regional network widely posted information about a woman who was killed as a consequence of GBV during the campaign itself.

As a direct result of the campaign, 18 women suffering from GBV came forward and sought help from Ma'an. Another 18 women were referred to Ma'an after hearing the radio spots aired during the campaign, and a further 10 came forward as a consequence of social media stories. Finally, 36 additional women were referred for legal assistance.

The steering committee for this campaign established by Ma'an, while composed of members of other CBOs, also included representatives of institutions from different villages and towns in the area. Representatives of the Ministries of Education and Welfare attended meetings as well. The committee met regularly and went beyond addressing the campaign to help strengthen the activities and the work of the regional network in general. Representatives of Ben Gurion University, located in the area, together with Kayan Feminist Organization, a former HATD grantee, also participated. Ma'an initiated workshops and seminars for professionals, including lawyers (with the assistance of the Ministry of Justice) and social workers. Representatives from the welfare departments in the targeted villages, the education department, and other CBOs held four meetings to discuss the campaign, feedback, and interaction and how to expand it to other villages in the Negev. The Ministry of Justice invited Ma'an leadership to conduct a roundtable session, which was attended by 21 people from the district attorney's office and the department of legal assistance. This steering committee and the entire campaign against GBV gave significant exposure to Ma'an's work, which increased the likelihood of sustainability for Ma'an's program after HATD's funding ended.

Summary of measurable objectives/outcomes

Objective: Sustainability of the work now that the third year is finished.

Outcome: Ma'an was able to secure funding to continue the work from the Global Fund for Women and UN Women. In addition, the Israeli Ministry of Labor, Social Affairs and Social Services will also continue to provide assistance. However, these commitments are neither settled nor secure, entailing an ongoing struggle to find support to fight against GBV among Bedouin women.

Objective: Increasing the awareness of women in the Negev of gender-based violence (GBV), mainly domestic violence.

Outcome: 388 women participated in a series of workshops encouraging them to become agents of change in their local communities. Focus group/questionnaire results: 29 women participated in five structured focus groups that included standardized questions. The number of participants was too small to draw statistically valid conclusions. However, focus group participants demonstrated increased understanding of gender-based abuse and issues affecting women's health. They all stated that they had gained very valuable skills and information. Many women who participated in the workshops conducted by Ma'an contacted the center for legal assistance and consultation.

Objective: Strengthening the capacities of the regional network of women focused on GBV

Outcome: The regional network continued its meetings and concentrated on the national campaign against GBV. In the final year, the regional network conducted 10 meetings that mainly consisted of training individuals in campaigning, advocacy, and mobilizing people to join the campaign. Ma'an plans to maintain the regional network; to this end, it has met with Kayan, a prior HATD grantee, to discuss the plan for regional network continuity. Kayan has its own regional women's network in the northern part of Israel called Juzoor.

Objective: Changing attitudes toward GBV in the Bedouin community

Outcome: Ma'an, together with the regional network, published a video as an awareness raiser on GBV. The video, titled *Discussion behind Masks*, attracted widespread attention and new engagement with Ma'an.

Discussion

Women and girls are among the most discriminated against people in the world. Gender-based violence—in particular, domestic violence—is the most reprehensible form of this discrimination (see also chapter 7). Fighting against GBV requires not just leadership but also personal bravery. Those who fight against GBV literally put their lives at risk. The work is even more challenging when seen through the lens of either the Israeli-Palestinian conflict or the discrimination suffered by the Bedouin in Israeli society.

Beyond expertly implementing a very challenging initiative, the leadership and staff of Ma'an were able to make the program, for now, sustainable. They managed to accomplish this with the engagement of HATD funds and expertise (particularly on the campaign), together with learning from other HATD grantees. While domestic violence will never be eradicated, initiatives such as that implemented by Ma'an using evidence-based approaches can make a significant dent in this worldwide problem. The sharing of successes and challenges with other HATD grantees of a societal problem impacted by an active conflict represents an integral part of peace building through health.

Appendix: qualitative anecdotes

1 After she heard about Ma'an services on the radio on the second day of the 16 Days of Activism Campaign against GBV, a transgender resident of a Bedouin village, then 39 years old, called the hotline. Her family members had isolated her, and she stated that she was lonely and subject to verbal violence and slander. She called to receive support and assistance from various health care institutions, as she wanted to undergo sex change surgery. Ma'an reached out to the organization al Qaws for Sexual & Gender Diversity in Palestinian Society, which arranged for the surgery. Ma'an continued providing this woman with psychological support and contacted the Ministry of Labor, Social Affairs and Social Services to find her a safe place to live, as her family threatened her life if she underwent the operation.

2 During one of the Ma'an workshops, a participant said that a cousin was sexually assaulting the participant's sister. After several conversations over the phone, she acknowledged that she, not her sister, was the victim, but she asked that her story not be shared with the Department of Social Affairs office in her village. As she was a minor (16 years old), Ma'an was legally obliged to inform the Department of Social Affairs, but with the girl's consent, instead informed the main office in Beersheva, not her village.

In coordination with the Ministry of Labor, Social Affairs and Social Services and the girl, Ma'an staff decided to file a police complaint. Ma'an staff were able to contact one of her uncles, again with her consent, who protected her and kept the aggressor away from her and her house. Personnel at Ma'an have maintained contact with the girl over the phone to support her and help her regain her confidence in herself.

3 AH, a social worker from Beersheva, a workshop participant: "I never thought that polygamy was a form of violence against women. After the first workshop, I went home thinking about it and today [the second workshop] I was thinking about this phenomenon and its implications on women. Thank you for opening my eyes to this specific issue and the violence against women in general. I thank you for all this valuable information that would help me in my career."

4 A fourth and last anecdote comes from the author (NG). For the past several years, HATD has sponsored a daylong meeting of our Israeli and Palestinian grantees. It is well attended, but some Palestinian grantees refuse to meet with Israeli grantees. There is no publicity surrounding the daylong meeting. At a recent meeting, I presented on stress and examined this issue in concentric circles starting with the individual, moving to the family, next to work (if the individual was working), then to the ethnic group or community, and finally to the nation. We broke into small groups to further discuss the concept of stress. One woman from Ma'an described her stress: My family doesn't know that I work at Ma'an. I do not know what they would do if they found out. I therefore just say that I am volunteering at a school.

Notes

1 Jewkes, R., (2002) Intimate partner violence: Causes and prevention. *Lancet.* 359 (9315), pp: 1423–1429.
2 UN Women. (2020) *Facts and Figures: Ending Violence against Women and Girls.* Available at: https://arabstates.unwomen.org/en/what-we-do/ending-violence-against-women/facts-and-figures; Accessed: June 17, 2020.
3 UN Women. (2020) *Families in A Changing World.* Available at: https://www.unwomen.org/en/digital-library/progress-of-the-worlds-women. Accessed: June 17, 2020.
4 Beeri, T. (2019) Israel shows no tolerance for violence against women. *The Jerusalem Post* https://www.jpost.com/Israel-News/Israel-shows-no-tolerance-for-violence-against-women-609002. Accessed: March 17, 2020.
5 Solomon, S. (2016) 40% of Israeli women aged 16-48 suffered partner violence – study. *The Times of Israel.* (https://www.timesofisrael.com/40-of-israeli-women-aged-16-48-suffered-partner-violence-study/ Accessed: March 17, 2020.
    Daoud, N., Sergienko, R., O'Campo, P., et al. (2017). Disorganization theory, neighborhood social capital, and ethnic inequalities in intimate partner violence between Arab and Jewish women citizens of Israel. *Journal of Urban Health 94*(5), pp: 648–665.
6 Daoud, N., Berger-Polsky, A., Sergienko, R., et al (2019). Screening and receiving information for intimate partner violence in healthcare settings: a cross-sectional study of Arab and Jewish women of childbearing age in Israel. *BMJ open*, *9*(2). Available at: https://www.ncbi.nlm.nih.gov/pmc/articles/PMC6398676/pdf/bmjopen-2018-022996.pdf. Accessed: June 17, 2020.
7 Note this is well before the COVID-19 pandemic.

Chapter 11

One in Nine

Community-based breast cancer initiatives

Norbert Goldfield

Introduction

In the Occupied Palestinian Territory (OPT), reports show that 70% of Palestinian women present with breast cancer in Stages III or IV.[1] It is difficult to ascertain mammography rates in the OPT with certainty, but limited research indicates that it is quite low.[2] Screening, diagnosis, treatment, and surveillance services also have significant opportunities for improvement.[3] Breast cancer is the most common form of cancer in Israeli women, accounting for nearly 30% of all new cancers.[4] In Israel, the incidence of breast cancer has been rising steadily since the late 1990s among Jewish and Palestinian women, with approximately 4,000 new cases diagnosed annually.[5] While rates of mammography and clinical breast exams (CBE) have improved since 2000, they remain lower among ultra-Orthodox Jewish and Palestinian women living in Israel as compared to, for example, non-religious Israeli Jewish women.[6]

This chapter summarizes two breast cancer interventions in Israel that HATD has sponsored since it was founded in 2004, together with efforts to implement a major breast cancer care intervention in the OPT. Some of the initiatives are just beginning, others were successful and adopted by major national organizations, and others remain to get off the ground. The first intervention in Israel to be discussed is the effort by Beit Natan, a community group based in Jerusalem, to increase rates of mammography and clinical breast exams (CBE) administered by female health practitioners among ultra-Orthodox Jewish women living in Jerusalem. The intervention, with the participation of an Israeli managed care organization (MCO) in the trial, was successful. Yet after the three years of funding ended, the MCO decided not to adopt the program. The second initiative that we funded was with another organization also focused on breast cancer, One in Nine, in conjunction with a partner, the Jewish Federation of Cleveland. The objective was again to increase mammography rates among ultra-Orthodox Jewish women. The intervention again worked, and this time, learning from the previous experience, we succeeded in persuading two of the principal MCOs in Israel to adopt this program.

Finally, HATD has spent considerable effort and resources on two—thus far, unsuccessful—attempts to implement a comprehensive approach to breast cancer diagnosis, treatment, and surveillance for Palestinian women. These initiatives were developed in conjunction with Italian breast cancer experts. In addition, major Italian cancer institutions have expressed their interest in participating. This chapter will summarize these two very different proposals developed five years apart and specify next steps in an effort to move forward a critical initiative that could measurably impact the lives of Palestinian women.

Beit Natan

The Israel Cancer Association and the Israeli HMOs promote the early detection of breast cancer through the practice of mammography and clinical breast examinations (CBE). The Israeli national health insurance law (which covers all Israeli citizens) does not pay for mammography screening for women under age 50, leaving women aged 30 to 49 vulnerable. While there is expert consensus that CBE should not be used as the only screening tool, there are medical societies that encourage it as an adjunctive tool.[7] In addition, although established research has shown a lack of benefit for breast self-examination (BSE), the World Health Organization recommends BSE as a way to empower and raise awareness among women.[8] However, there are an insufficient number of examiners to perform CBE, the majority of whom are male (at the time of this initiative, only surgeons were allowed to perform CBE). Traditional and religious beliefs of both Jewish and Palestinian women have inhibited most religious women from undergoing the exam performed by male practitioners. In 2007, Beit Natan embarked on a three-year project to rectify this gap in health care, targeting its pilot program to the traditional/modest populations in the Bayit Vagan neighborhood of Jerusalem.

Beit Natan is a Jerusalem-based organization that focuses on the health of Haredi (ultra-Orthodox) and Orthodox Jewish women and on increasing women's awareness of their responsibility to take care of their physical and emotional health. Specifically, the objectives of this project were to:

- train female physicians from all four HMOs in a standardized CBE method and to analyze their subsequent delivery of the CBE in the community setting for ease of delivery and physician confidence in the method;
- encourage an increase in Haredi women's compliance with CBE.

Methodology and results

In the initial project year, Beit Natan staff contacted community leaders and teachers (bridal teachers, mikvah [Orthodox Jewish ritual baths for women] attendants, health care professionals) and asked them, in turn, to reach out to their customer base of Haredi women. In 2008–9, the emphasis was on reaching and training professionals with the goal of increasing the number of female doctors performing CBE. Fourteen female physicians (family practitioners and gynecologists) participated in a ten-hour training session in performance of CBE in year 1. Each woman physician received 10 hours of apprenticeship, totaling 140 hours of breast exam training conducted in the community. From March through June 2009, 560 women received CBEs. Additional early detection lectures and direct waiting room solicitation yielded the examinations of 84 more women.

A second nonprofit organization utilized Beit Natan's training concept and recruited another 12 physicians for its training. For the second training, Beit Natan decided to partner with Kupat Holim Meuhedet and Kupat Holim Leumit, two large managed care organizations (MCOs) that serve the religious populations (both Arab and Jewish) of Jerusalem, and requested that they recruit their physicians. Other trainings were implemented.

According to Beit Natan's final report: "What cannot be quantified but which is an additional accomplishment of this training is the dissemination of Beit Natan's mission in the medical community through this training." As a result of the HATD-funded initiative, 150 female physicians in Jerusalem were trained in CBE. While the leadership of the two MCOs Leumit and Meuhedet were aware of Beit Natan's activities and successes, no MCO decided to adopt the Beit Natan approach of encouraging female health professional breast care of ultra-Orthodox Jewish women. It required another HATD-funded initiative in this arena for Israeli MCOs to take notice of and adopt a community-based breast wellness intervention benefiting the Orthodox Jewish population.

One in Nine and two Israeli MCOs

This second initiative ran from 2012 to 2014. Joint funding was provided by HATD and the Jewish Federation of Cleveland. (More details on this partnership, which lasted several years, can be found in chapter 15.) This breast cancer initiative was similar in many ways to the Beit Natan intervention described above. One in Nine, a national not-for-profit organization based in Israel, "strives to raise public awareness of breast cancer and advance breast health in Israel, including by means of public campaigns and via workshops for the early detection of breast cancer." The One in Nine intervention had the following objectives:

- to increase the number of ultra-Orthodox (Haredi) women who undergo mammography;
- to increase the awareness of the importance of early detection among the professional teams in the MCOs and the creation of a leadership committed to this issue.

A unique element of this intervention was that HATD signed a legal agreement with One in Nine and one of the Israeli MCOs participating in the initiative obligating the MCO to adopt the intervention if successful.

The intervention featured the following activities:

- training medical teams of Leumit (family doctors, nurses, and medical secretaries) to raise awareness of the importance of early detection of the disease and to help them convince Orthodox women to undergo mammography;
- workshops for Orthodox women to raise awareness of the importance of early detection and mammography tests. This was done in conjunction with community health workers (called advocates);
- communication with important stakeholders, such as rabbis and rebbetzin (wives of rabbis), in the community and obtaining their endorsement wherever possible.

Summary results from the One in Nine final report

Increase in response rates for mammography: The mammography rate increased 1.9% in Leumit centers that did not implement the intervention and 7.59% in those that did. The denominator was in the tens of thousands, though the precise number was never specified.

Creating and strengthening of trust in One in Nine among the Haredi community: Leading Haredi organizations viewed One in Nine as an authoritative organization for teaching health content and workshops in their community. This became evident in increased name recognition, which was apparent during interviews, and more invitations for activities (Citybook Services, a company that employs Haredi women in Jerusalem, invited One in Nine to give the workshop in its office).

Approval of One in Nine's action by rabbis: This was an important achievement, as breast health is an extremely taboo subject among the Haredi population in Israel. One in Nine approached several rabbis regarding mammography and received signatures on an updated ruling from rabbis involved with the Refuah Institute, an organization that provides Torah-based medical diplomas and certificates to members of the Haredi community. The rabbinical approvals were sent to family doctors, regional managers, nurses, and Leumit medical secretaries to be placed on the branch message boards in order to encourage Haredi women to undergo mammography.

In addition, a meeting was held with Rabbi Chananya Chollack, CEO of Ezer Mizion (an Israeli health support organization offering a wide range of medical and social support services for Israel's sick, disabled, and elderly), and he expressed an interest in helping One in Nine reach leading influential rabbis in the Haredi sector throughout Israel. A very supportive senior rabbi who had lost his wife to breast cancer also joined the effort. In short, involving rabbis, their wives, and leaders in the religious communities of Israel is a long process, but with their support, health initiatives such as this one have a chance of success.

Strengthened relationship with mammography centers: One in Nine established tight contracts with Mayanei Hayeshua Hospital, which serves the Haredi population in Bnei Brak and has centers in Jerusalem (Mar Center) and Netanya (Mammography Center). This strengthened Leumit's relationship with these centers and made the programs more accessible to women in terms of availability and location.

Increased trust with *kupot* (MCOs): Establishing trust with Leumit was a fundamental aspect of this project, as it required Leumit to transfer sensitive information and allowed an outside organization, One in Nine, to be part of the doctor-patient relationship. The manager of Leumit's Central District, Dr. Avivit Golan, and its national health promotion manager, Margalit Shilo, both claimed that the project resonated throughout the entire HMO and has influenced additional Haredi branches where One in Nine has not been active, as well as branches serving other demographics. In fact, after this initiative ended, two Israeli MCOs, Leumit and Meuhedet, adopted the One in Nine program.

Cooperation with HATD grantee organizations: One in Nine cooperated with the Yasmin Organization (a prior HATD grantee) and the Community Centers Network (another HATD grantee). Together with Yasmin, One in Nine wrote a proposal to raise awareness of the importance of early detection breast cancer and increase the accessibility to examinations for Bedouin women in the Negev area. One in Nine also established a strong alliance with the Community Centers Network, participating in activities taking place in the Haredi community in Har Nof.

Challenges, difficulties, insights, and lessons

Barriers that hinder Orthodox women from undergoing early detection tests:

Questionnaires circulated by One in Nine revealed the following attitudes:

- lack of knowledge and awareness of the disease and methods of prevention;
- mammography is painful;
- belief that there is no reason to be tested if there is no pain and no interference with normal life;
- modesty makes use of the word "breast" uncommon;
- women are concentrated on family life and avoid long-term planning; they do not set appointments;
- women are afraid of finding out about the BRCA 1/2 gene, as it might make their daughters less "marriageable."

Activity with health advocates: Through this initiative, One in Nine learned that health advocates are the main agents of change in the Haredi community. They all come into direct contact with the patients on a daily basis. In the Jerusalem District, medical secretaries were recruited as health advocates, and in the Central District, One in Nine recruited nurses. The advantage in selecting nurses as advocates is that they are more proficient in medical issues and better understand the importance of mammography than others; they also have higher credibility among patients and physicians. The main disadvantage to working with nurses, however, is their already high workload and lack of availability. One in Nine added two Haredi volunteers in Bnei Brak to make phone calls to patients and also trained medical secretaries in Netanya. These changes increased the rate of women who underwent mammography in these locations. One in Nine therefore hired 10 more volunteers, as well as proposed to Leumit that medical secretaries or phone operators should be utilized.

Implementation highlighted the need to encourage the use of health advocates. It is important to note that the advocates did not receive additional time to work on the project or additional compensation for performing the required tasks. Thus, One in Nine:

1 Encouraged Leumit to find a way to compensate them. Leumit decided to award monetary prizes for exceptional advocates;
2 Held personal supervision meetings with health advocates in order to increase motivation and clarify needs, goals, and objectives of the program. In branches where these meetings were held, substantial change was observed.
3 Trained advocates to teach seminars (training the trainers). This gave them the opportunity to become more professional and knowledgeable in the field of breast health, which, in turn, further motivates and enables advocates to coordinate workshops on their own. The training allows them to work as instructors both inside and outside the MCOs, thus creating a viable career track. An additional advantage in employing advocates as instructors is that the MCOs are able to continue the activity after the project ends.

Media exposure: Media outreach is critical. However, One in Nine encountered difficulties in advertising through Haredi channels. The main challenge is that the Haredi media do not permit the use of words such as "cancer" or "breast" (in newspapers or on the radio). The media do not publish images of women; and most radio stations do not allow women on the air. In the general media, One in Nine encountered challenges trying to convince Haredi women to share their experiences or images of themselves, as they harbor fears of public exposure and victimization. Eventually, two Haredi newspapers published announcements regarding early detection, and the mainstream newspaper *Maariv* covered the story. The stories were different, as the former, reflecting ideals of "modesty," did not mention "breast cancer" specifically, just "cancer."

Concluding comments

This three-year partnership with the Jewish Federation of Cleveland had a significant capacity-building impact on the grantee, One in Nine, and increased the mammography rates of the women served. The two MCOs that signed the initial agreement adopted the model and integrated the model into ongoing operations. HATD facilitated meetings with other Israeli HATD grantees, resulting in cooperative initiatives between One in Nine with both Jewish and Palestinian Israeli grantees.

Initiatives to improve breast cancer care among Palestinian women in the OPT

Twice since 2015, Healing Across the Divides pursued two major initiatives to improve breast cancer services for Palestinian women living in the OPT. In 1996, when I first began to work as a clinician in the OPT village of Biddu near Ramallah, I read a report issued by Physicians for Human Rights Israel entitled "A Death Foretold." It told the story of a Palestinian woman from Gaza with breast cancer who encountered obstacle after obstacle in obtaining appropriate care. She died within a year of her diagnosis.[9]

There are many obstacles to breast cancer care in the OPT. Many have documented the challenges, most recently, Physicians for Human Rights Israel and Medical Aid to Palestine. To begin with, there is only one hospital, Augusta Victoria Hospital in East Jerusalem, that provides radiation therapy for the entire OPT, which means that patients have to travel through checkpoints.[10]

In 2014, HATD worked with Augusta Victoria Hospital (represented by the then-CEO Tawfiq Nasser) and a team of three breast cancer experts from Italy (Giovanni Apolone, MD, Giorgio Mazzi, MD, Pierpaolo Pattacini, MD) and United Nations Relief and Works Agency (UNRWA, headed by Dr. Seita, head of UNRWA for the Middle East). We met with the Palestinian Authority Ministry of Health (MoH), the American consulate in Jerusalem, and other organizations. These meetings were supplemented by other information gathered by the entire team of individuals represented by the above organizations. The overall objective of these meetings was to develop a proposal to implement breast cancer screening, detection, diagnosis, and treatment among Palestinian women living in the territory administered by the Palestinian Authority (PA), with hoped-for dissemination eventually to Gaza, at that point administered by Hamas.

The following summarizes the recommendations of this first breast cancer proposal:

a **Consolidation** of Breast Cancer services into three Ministry of Health centers of excellence for breast cancer care: centers covering the North, Central, and Southern parts of the West Bank administered by the Palestinian Authority.

b An **epidemiological (Web-based) tracking system**. The Italian team offered training opportunities for establishing such a system.

c **Mammography**: The Italian team pointed to the necessity of 5,000 cases read per year per radiologist as the European standard. The Italian team offered training opportunities.

d Training in **fine needle biopsies**.

e **Sentinel lymph node biopsies:** No radioactive tracers, essential for carrying out this test, are available in MoH institutions in part because of security reasons. The Italian team offered training opportunities and access to tracers.

f **Surgery** is done in many private centers with little training. The hospital at Beit Jalla is the only hospital performing lumpectomies and quadrantectomies. The Italian team offered training opportunities.

g **Biomarkers:** For financial reasons, biomarkers are available only for specific subgroups of women and only for a few months at a time. The Italian team offered the possibility of obtaining these biomarkers.

h **Radiation therapy** is performed only at Augusta Victoria Hospital (AVH). While the services are available, radiation therapy is performed in a timely fashion at best in 60% of all cases. Delays, which can be a month or more, are largely related to security issues. Medical physics is not available anywhere except for AVH. The Italian team offered training opportunities.

i **Chemotherapy:** There are different courses of chemotherapy, and not all are available. The Italian team offered opportunities for a regular supply of chemotherapy.

j A **post-treatment surveillance program** does not appear to be well established in the PA. The Italian team offered training opportunities to set up such a program.

Despite many meetings and the availability of funds for the initiative, no project ensued, for reasons that are not clear to me.

Tawfiq Nasser, the CEO of AVH, enthusiastically supported the effort and came to many meetings but was dubious about the likelihood of the MoH adopting the program. His judgment proved correct. The opportunity for this important initiative lay dormant until 2019.

In March 2019, during our annual HATD Study Tour, I asked a local Palestinian female in Nablus, after establishing rapport with her, if she had ever had a mammogram. She said absolutely not and would never do so. Her sister had died of breast cancer and received poor care in Palestinian hospitals. Her other sister was actually dying of breast cancer.

The interaction with this Palestinian woman prompted me to re-explore opportunities for engagement with the Palestinian Ministry of Health on a breast cancer initiative. Instead of a national approach, I explored the possibility of implementing a comprehensive breast cancer program in one province or governorate. The proposal was developed in conjunction with the Azienda Unita Sanitaria Locale di Reggio Emilia. Azienda Reggio Emilia and Healing Across the Divides suggested focusing on the district of Jenin. Our analysis projected 21,000 eligible women; 8,000 mammograms; 300 biopsies; and 15–20 breast cancer cases.

The proposed work is intended as a pilot effort to determine the opportunities for improvement in screening, diagnosis, treatment, and surveillance in Palestine. If the Palestinian Ministry of Health is interested, Palestinian and other experts will determine actual resource needs for breast cancer care in a Palestinian district. This second proposal to address breast cancer in Palestinian women is still in negotiation.

Concluding comments

Thus far we've been successful in the community-based breast cancer initiatives that we funded in Israel. In addition, we learned from the first initiative how to prepare the ground to integrate the initiative, once it proved successful, into parts of the Israeli health system.

In contrast, our much more ambitious efforts in the OPT have not come to fruition. Why not? In part, the Palestinian proposals simply placed the bar too high. More than just trying to encourage early detection, as was done in the two Israeli initiatives, we were trying to address the entire pathway of breast cancer care. Such an ambition goes beyond the problems of a much more complex clinical undertaking, since any complex clinical set of interventions implies engagement with local economic and political interests. We were and are hoping to work with the Palestinian Ministry of Health (MoH). However, we recognize that while in theory, the MoH has responsibility for all aspects of breast care, in practice, it faces considerable organizational, practical, and financial challenges.

It should be emphasized that funders have spent considerable monies on the different aspects of breast cancer care, such as mammography machines. However, while USAID, the European Union, foundations, and other aid agencies have been willing to fund screening interventions in the OPT, none of these interventions has taken a comprehensive perspective or made a significant effort to perform follow-up research to ascertain that the intervention was sustainable. This is especially important in the OPT, which, in contrast to Israel or the United States, has no centralized health system. As discussed in the last chapter, HATD will intensify its pursuit of these national efforts in the OPT, complex as they may be, as part of our future strategy of explicitly fostering community-based interventions that have the clear potential for changes at the national level.

Personal note

The most gratifying part of creating and leading Healing Across the Divides is our engagement with the leaders of the community groups that we fund and work with. Here, I would like to highlight one individual: Chaya Heller, the founder of Beit Natan. She is just one of many amazing women that I've met since 2004. Sadly, she passed away in 2011, way too soon.

The following is an excerpt from a recommendation for an award I wrote on her behalf. It conveys the spirit of some of the women I've been fortunate to meet with since founding Healing Across the Divides. I am particularly happy that my daughter had the opportunity to meet Chaya Heller.

Dear Recommendation Committee,

I knew Ms. Chaya Heller, the nominee, for approximately ten years. She was, simply put, a force for change—both for her family and for the Haredi women she sought to assist. As executive director of Healing Across the Divides, I knew Ms. Heller for the amazing work that she did, on issues pertaining to breast cancer. In the last five years, Chaya began a new project, and I had the privilege of working with her. She realized that in order to be successful at changing the health perceptions of the women, we needed to modify the perceptions of the physicians and the health-care policy makers. She was acutely aware of this because during her pregnancy with her fifth daughter, Chaya was diagnosed with multiple sclerosis, a disease that accompanied her throughout the rest of her life.

Walking into a room with Chaya was always an experience. I'm not sure what people expected when she would enter, a woman dressed in typical Haredi fashion, with a wig, a pronounced limp, sometimes with a cane, and always with a bright, sharp smile. She was incredibly forthright, honest, and clear. She never minced words. Chaya believed strongly in what she was doing and managed to infect others with that belief. Those who worked with her, from the health funds, the physicians in the hospitals, to the funders, were her lifelong advocates after just a brief time with her.

Chaya Heller dedicated her life to helping women: mothers, daughters, sisters, all who were suffering from illness or supporting someone who was ill or preventing illness from happening. She was there. Even on her deathbed, she was reviewing applications for a future grant. Chaya Heller passed away recently. Even as I write this recommendation, I have tears in my eyes. I knew Chaya as a colleague, a mentor, a grantee recipient. I did not realize how much I would miss her when she was gone. Her legacy lives on in the actions of Beit Natan, whose staff continues her work, and through her five children.

An excerpt from her autobiography: "We are all snowflakes, falling from the sky, landing, and making our unique impact during our short existence in this lifetime. My snowflake journey continues to be transformative. It is this physical and spiritual journey that I wish to share with you."

She did not get the recognition she deserved in her lifetime. Please honor her family and her legacy with this recognition in her death.

Sincerely,
Norbert Goldfield, M.D.

Notes

1 Breast cancer in occupied Palestine (2016) Available at: http://www.phr.org.il/wp-content/uploads/2016/10/MAPPFHR-Breast-Cancer-fact-sheet-WEB.pdf. Accessed: June 20, 2020.

2 Ibid.

3 Halahleh, K., Gale, R.K. (2018) Cancer care in the Palestinian territories. *The Lancet Oncology* 19(7), pp. E359–E369.

4 Israel Cancer Association (2020) *Breast Cancer.* Available at: https://en.cancer.org.il/template_e/default.aspx?PageId=7749. Accessed: June 20, 2020.

5 Ibid.

6 Tkatch, R., Hudson, J., Katz, A., et al (2014). Barriers to cancer screening among orthodox Jewish women. *Journal of Community Health, 39*(6), pp: 1200–1208.

7 Practice Bulletin Number 179: (2017) Breast cancer risk assessment and screening in average-risk women. Committee on Practice Bulletins—*Gynecology Obstet Gynecol.* p: 130(1):e1.

8 World Health Organization, (2012) Awareness is the first step in battle against breast cancer. *Bulletin of the World Health Organization* 90(3) Available at: https://www.who.int/bulletin/volumes/90/3/12-030312/en/. Accessed: February 2021.

9 Bendel, M. (2005) Breast cancer in the Gaza strip: a death foretold dedicated with love to the memory of Fattum; Physicians for Human Rights-Israel. As quoted in Al Waheidi, S. (2019) Breast cancer in Gaza—a public health priority in search of reliable data. *E Cancer Medical Science,* pp: 1–8. Available at: file:///C:/Users/Rin83/Downloads/Breast_cancer_in_Gaza-a_public_health_priority_in_.pdf. Accessed: June 20, 2020.

10 Medical aid for Palestinians, physicians for human rights, Israel. (2018) *Breast Cancer in Occupied Palestine.* Available at: https://www.map.org.uk/downloads/map-breast-cancer-in-opt-2018-online.pdf. Accessed: June 29, 2020.

Chapter 12

Palestinian Working Women Society for Development

Building resilience in the Hebron Hills in Occupied Palestinian Territory

Norbert Goldfield

Introduction

This chapter highlights the engagement of Healing Across the Divides (HATD) with a Palestinian grantee, the Palestinian Working Women Society for Development (PWWSD). The PWWSD, utilizing funding and technical/managerial advice from HATD, provides counseling and social/awareness-building services to women and, primarily, teenage girls in the South Hebron Hills in the Occupied Palestinian Territory (OPT), an area under total Israeli security and administrative control. Many of their communities, neighborhoods, homes are under orders of demolition. These services relate to an overall effort by PWWSD to build psychological resilience among the Palestinian residents of the South Hebron Hills of the West Bank (see the map in Appendix 1 for the location of Susiya and surrounding villages).

The chapter includes a brief description of the overall initiative, consisting largely of qualitative data drawn from focus groups and individual clients. In addition, it summarizes efforts on the part of HATD staff to engage with American public officials in an effort to protect the villages from demolition.

The setting

Since the first intifada of 1989, Israelis and Palestinians have fought with each other in a variety of major "uprisings" against the Israeli occupation of Palestinian territories, or intifadas, in combination with ongoing outbursts of violence against Israeli occupation that occur on a regular basis in Gaza, Israel, or the West Bank. After Israel won the 1967 war against the surrounding Arab countries, Israel occupied the West Bank and Gaza. This defeat is what the Palestinians call Al Naksa.[1] Following the signing of the Oslo Accords in 1993, the West Bank was divided into three zones: A, B, and C (see Appendix 1 for map). Area A (approximately 18% of the West Bank) is nominally under the control of the Palestinian Authority (PA), although the Israeli military conducts regular incursions into this territory. It contains the major cities in the West Bank, including Hebron, Jenin, Nablus, and Ramallah. Area B (about 22%) is in theory jointly administered by the Israeli military authority and the Palestinian Authority. Area C (about 60%), the vast majority of the land of the West Bank, is administered by the Israeli military authority. The majority of Palestinian agricultural land is located in Area C. Many Palestinians live in Area C, under very difficult circumstances, and have to go through an extensive permit process to build any homes or dig wells. The PWWSD initiative is situated in Area C.

The PWWSD initiative has taken place in Palestinian communities called *khirab* south of Hebron and near the southern border of the West Bank with Israel. The *khirab* (plural of *khirbet*, meaning "small community") are geographically smaller than villages, and their populations include only a few hundred people. Khirbet Susiya, which originated in the early nineteenth century, is one of these small Palestinian *khirab*/communities.[2] For this initiative, the PWWSD focused its efforts on Susiya, but it also worked in other villages, including Twaneh, al-Fakheet, and Masafer Yatta.

In 1983, the Israeli Jewish settlement of Susiya was established near the khirbet, on Palestinian land that had been declared state land by Israel. In 1986, about twenty-five Palestinian families were living in Khirbet Susiya, in caves and structures. That year, the Israeli Civil Administration declared the khirbet's land an "archaeological site"; the land was confiscated "for public purposes" and the Israeli military expelled its residents from their homes. Having no other option, the families relocated to other caves in the area and to flimsy wood-frame shelters and tents they erected on agricultural land a few hundred meters southeast of the original village and the archaeological site. The military expelled the residents again several times after 1986, including once in 2001 after a Palestinian killed an Israeli Jewish resident of the Susiya settlement.

Residents of Susiya have been embroiled in legal battles with the Israeli state for decades. Most recently, in late 2017 the Israeli Supreme Court ruled that the Israeli army may proceed to demolish the entire village of Susiya. As of this writing this has not yet occurred. In February 2018, the latest demolition order was handed down to the residents of Susiya; the Israeli High Court of Justice decided that seven structures in the village of Susiya could be demolished by Israel without delay. These seven structures are home to 42 residents of the village, of which half are children. Jihad Nawajaa, 49, the head of the local village council, said, "Every day we wait; we wait for the Israeli bulldozers to come." He added: "Can you imagine the psychological effects this has on the people, on the children, who are always wondering when the next demolition order or settler attack will come?"[3]

Palestinian Working Women Society for Development (PWWSD) is a Palestinian women's rights organization founded in 1981. The organization believes that liberating women is connected directly with ending the Israeli occupation and establishing a Palestinian democratic sovereign civil state. PWWSD operates all over the West Bank, including East Jerusalem, as well as in the Gaza Strip and is an active member in several local, regional, and global networks and coalitions, such as the Palestinian NGO Network, the Arab Women Network (Aisha), Women National Coalition for the implementation of UNSCR 1325, Karama network, and the International Union for Workers Education, among others.

Methods

The interventions of the PWWSD in several villages in the South Hebron Hills consisted of the following: awareness-raising/empowerment sessions for teenage girls and their mothers; debriefing sessions for teachers; well-being sessions for parents and children; individual sessions with children and adults; and a media campaign. With the technical assistance of HATD (evaluation assistance in particular provided by Lewis Kazis, Boston University School of Public Health, and Elizabeth Hembree, University of Pennsylvania), evaluations of the intervention were done largely through focus groups, in lieu of responses to written questionnaires. Illiteracy and cultural constraints (fear of being identified through questionnaire completion) did not allow for the collection of valid information from written questionnaires. All counselors and individuals working directly on the project were from the South Hebron Hills, the geographic area of the intervention. The leadership of the PWWSD is based in Ramallah, in the center of the West Bank.

In addition, in year 2 of this three-year grant, Professor Elizabeth Hembree of the University of Pennsylvania, under the aegis of HATD, conducted a three-day program for 25 therapists from throughout the West Bank in treatment approaches to post-traumatic stress disorder (PTSD). Subsequent to this intensive training, Professor Hembree led one-hour therapy review sessions, during which PWWSD counselors could bring up challenging therapeutic situations.

HATD has an annual study tour in which we visit HATD grantees such as PWWSD in Susiya. After they returned home, some study tour participants have engaged with American elected officials regarding issues pertaining to Susiya.

Results

By way of examples, the PWWSD conducted the following types of sessions in the third year with the women and teenage girls in the South Hebron Hills villages:

a   Awareness-raising/empowerment sessions for teenage girls and mothers: many sessions, with 10–15 people in each session; 235 participants.
b   Debriefing sessions for teachers.
c   Well-being sessions for parents and children: 110 participants.
d   Individual sessions with children and adults: 63 participants.

Similar kinds and numbers of sessions took place in the first two years of the grant. The PWWSD, utilizing a questionnaire co-developed with HATD consultants' expert in the development of evaluation instruments, posed the questions to focus groups (see Appendix 2 for more detailed results). In response to the question (translated from Arabic), "How did the workshops affect building your personal capacities?" Nasreen, a participant, answered, "We and our children feel frightened as a result of being continuously exposed to violations by Israeli soldiers and settlers like detention, assault and physical inspection, let alone the emotional and mental damage caused by the news over media channels. Therefore, workshops are important because they help us deal with our personal and family daily life pressures, and also increase awareness of new topics and issues such as different forms of violence, electronic violations and communication with our children—which is of utmost importance." (See Appendix 2 for the anecdotes derived from the questionnaire applied in a focus-group setting.)

Following are excerpts of quotes from young focus-group participants:

> Hamza, a male student: "I feel happy whenever I go out herding the sheep, so when I feel nervous and unhappy, I go out and start talking to my sheep, I have a baby sheep and I love it the most." Wissam, a male student, announced, "I will be in a vocational school because I want to learn how to build real strong houses for the people in my community." Most of the students agreed that they must tell their teachers and parents when they are subjected to violence. One of them said that when he sees the settlers coming his way, he runs away until he reaches the school or his house, whatever is closer to him. Bissan, a Palestinian student, commented that "since we are away from people, we prefer being in groups and going to school or home in groups, this way, we can defend each other when the settlers come." (See Appendix 2 for a more in-depth focus on one family.)

Though the PWWSD planned to have at least 75 children in the three debriefing sessions, only 44 attended, reflecting the tenuous political situation. The session was implemented during February 2018, a critical month during which the Israeli Supreme Court approved a demolition order to destroy the houses of Susiya. This had a major impact on the lives of people there, especially children. According to the teachers at Susiya, they witnessed a decrease in children's attendance at school as well. The settlers' attacks increased during this period, in an effort to spread fear among the people of Susiya.[4] (Recently, the Israeli Supreme Court reaffirmed the demolition order of Susiya).[5]

Other challenges affecting participation included harvest time, which limited the involvement of women, the holy month of Ramadan, a teacher's strike that lasted for more than two months during the second year of the grant, and bureaucratic barriers from the Palestinian Ministry of Education. Moreover, the aluminium-sheet roofs of the classrooms at Susiya made conducting meetings during extremely hot or cold weather stressful, thus discouraging women from attending the meetings.

Impact of the initiative on the PWWSD

PWWSD declared that the support of HATD, along with contributions from other partners, has enabled the continuity of its work at the grassroots level. Given the reality of the shrinking space of civil society, it remains challenging for organizations like PWWSD to maintain sustainability. The partnership with HATD is enriching the PWWSD organizationally. Externally, as a result of the continuous engagement between PWWSD staff and the Palestinian Authority (PA) Ministry of Education, the PWWSD was able to convince Ministry staff to have a part-time counselor available at Susiya's school, an important aspect of long-term sustainability for this effort. According to the PWWSD, this development has had a significant impact on students' academic performance, as reported by the school principal and the teachers. In addition, the PWWSD worked with the PA Ministry of Agriculture to plant trees in order to beautify the area of Susiya and to strengthen the resilience of the people on their land.

Media campaigns

In year 2, radio interviews were broadcast on topics and terminologies related to social and psychological health. These radio interviews were conducted twice a month for six months. In year 3, the PWWSD produced a radio spot and two brochures. The spot, a dramatized account based on a true story, covered the issue of early marriage and school dropout for girls, featuring one girl who talks about her experience in getting engaged at an early age (between 15 and 16) and is subjected to abuse by her fiancé and family for wanting to go back to school. They forced her to drop out. At the end of the spot, the girl goes back to school with the help of the counselor at PWWSD and leaves her fiancé. The radio piece aimed to convey that early marriage is a crime against childhood and that the rule of law should be enforced to protect children's right to a proper education. The two brochures, on "Adolescence" and "Psychological trauma," were suggested by the counselors based on the level of interest shown and the number of questions brought up by the participants (both children and parents) during the awareness-raising sessions and the individual consultations on these topics.

Engagements with American elected officials

Every year HATD leads a study tour of approximately 20 individuals. In response to the ongoing threat to demolish the entire village of Susiya, many of the HATD Study Tour participants have written letters to their US senators and representatives such as the one reproduced in Appendix 3.

Discussion/conclusion

It is difficult to evaluate these types of interventions, as the outcome we are seeking is increased individual and group strength and resilience on the part of the local population. Besides the major complication of the ongoing conflict, issues of cultural discomfort and lack of literacy pose significant barriers to reliable evaluation. Practical challenges added to the problems of implementing this work, such as military checkpoints that would delay appointments. Before starting their field visits to the villages, the counselors had to check the security situation. Additional delays were caused by the presence of temporary, or "flying," checkpoints. During the days when the counselors knew there were temporary checkpoints, they left earlier than usual to get to the villages they were visiting to conduct the sessions.

Despite these many logistical and political challenges, the PWWSD, utilizing funding and technical/managerial advice from HATD, accomplished its intermediate goals of building resilience and emotional strength among Palestinian women and teenage girls in the villages in the South Hebron Hills. The stories gathered through questionnaires, focus groups, and interviews with individuals that we have summarized provide anecdotal evidence of success. It must be emphasized that we were not able to collect numerical results from questionnaires; focus-group information reported in this chapter was drawn from the counselors. At the same time, the HATD representative made regular site visits to validate in a qualitative manner with villagers themselves the work that PWWSD counselors and staff were implementing.

At the most fundamental outcome level, Palestinians living in Susiya and surrounding villages have refused Israeli buyout offers and have remained in their homes while continuing to withstand settler harassment and awaiting very likely demolition of their homes. It is impossible to measure with any certainty to what extent the intervention documented in this chapter contributed to Palestinian determination to remain in place.

In November 2006, Human Rights Watch (HRW) produced the report "A Question of Security: Violence against Palestinian Women and Girls."[6] This extensively documented report on the challenges that women and girls face in the West Bank and Gaza contained recommendations for all levels of the Palestinian government (such as the judiciary and police). HRW also made specific recommendations for Israeli government/military authorities. Some of these might appear on the surface as fundamental or simple needs, such as: "Provide travel permits valid for use in times of closure to judges and other persons essential to the functioning of the Palestinian justice system. Instruct Israeli security personnel to honor such permits at checkpoints and facilitate passage."

HRW also recommended the following for NGOs such as HATD: "Provide capacity building for local professionals and enhance the use of local experts as much as possible in all donor-funded training and projects." HATD aspires to accomplish this and more in the South Hebron Hills. In short, with PWWSD, we aimed to help local communities in the South Hebron Hills in their struggle against the attempt to demolish their communities. This chapter demonstrates that Healing Across the Divides and the Palestinian Working Women Society for Development are striving, both in this initiative and our current ongoing separate work, to reach this objective, daunting as it may be.

Appendix 1: Map of the West Bank showing areas **A**, **B**, and **C**

Image © B'TSelem

Area A: Build Up Palestinian Area – Dark Brown
   Area A: Palestinian Control – Medium Brown
   Area B: Lightest Brown – Palestinian Civil (e.g. health, education) control
   Area C: Built up Jewish Settlement (Dark Blue)
   Area C: Area within Jewish Municipal Boundary (Moderate Blue)
   Area C: Jewish Regional Council Area (Light Blue)
   Area C: Israeli Control: (White)

   Grey line: Road
   Green line: 1949 Armistice Line also called the Green Line
   Purple Line: Approved "wall" or "fence" route
   Solid red line: Built Israeli "wall" or "fence"
   Broken red line: To be built Israeli 'wall" or "fence"

   Circle with orange color: Susiya, location of HATD intervention: Area C: Israeli control

Appendix 2: Evaluation of the community awareness workshops

Workshop topics: Nervousness, forgetfulness, sexual harassment through social networks, bed-wetting, violence against women, fear among children, exams anxiety, school underachievement, personal hygiene, development of self-control skills, psychological debriefing that helps to deal with life pressures, and coping mechanisms.

Evaluation methodology and participants: The evaluation adopted a focus-group methodology and targeted 10 women from Twaneh. The discussion addressed a number of questions, as follows:

- **First question: What is your knowledge and understanding of PWWSD's goals?**
  The group expressed a good level of knowledge about PWWSD's goals, services, target groups, and the counseling and empowerment programs. They were also aware of the confidentiality promised within PWWSD counseling services and were willing to have excerpts of their responses externally reported to HATD and used in additional reports such as scientific articles.

- **Second question: How do you feel you have benefited from attending the awareness workshops?**

The quotations below express the impact of the workshops on women as they explain in their own words:

> "The awareness workshops were of vital importance as they helped us develop strategies for self-understanding and self-control. They also acquainted us with new methods for becoming capable of dealing with our children's behavior and problems."

> "Even if we have experience and knowledge of these matters, human beings are continually acquiring new knowledge; this is why refreshing and renewing information is necessary."

> "It ... [the workshop] helps us understand how to deal with our children at different stages of their lives, in addition to looking for entertaining methods which develop their abilities and life skills."

> "I gained new information and knowledge. Moreover, my self-confidence and self-control have increased."

> "We have the ability to deal with others and with our life pressures.... Now I realize how to deal with people."

> "I am more aware of how to deal with people."

> "Increasing my self-confidence is very important for me; now I speak with confidence and I do not hesitate while making decisions."

> "The workshops steered my interest toward education; now I feel a burning desire for knowledge acquisition, and that ultimately reshaped my plans for future education."

> "What attracted my attention was the specific topic on how to protect myself against electronic violations across social media networks, the proper and safe usage for those networks, and the ability to transfer this knowledge to people in order to improve their self-protection."

> "The topic on abuse is new for us; now we have the ability to distinguish between the concepts of assault, rape and harassment. We acquired new methods of protecting ourselves against mistreatment."

> "Before the workshops we used to have a problem in coping with life difficulties. When the topics were presented in the first meeting, we did not have high expectations, but the current results show the importance of the workshops and

awareness whether for ourselves or in the way we deal with our children and others."

- **Third question: What are the new skills you acquired throughout the workshops, especially by working in groups?**
  The participants declared that they had acquired a set of skills that included self-confidence, self-expression, respect for others' opinions, self-defense mechanisms, and mechanisms for building social relations. These specific skills were identified based on the dynamic interaction and exchange of thoughts and experiences among participants during group work. Brainstorming also had a key role in refreshing the participants' information and encouraging them to talk about their personal experiences and the way they deal with life pressures and difficult conditions.
- **Fourth question: How did the workshops affect building your personal capacities?**
  When the participants were asked about the impact of the workshops on capacity building, they emphasized that they had developed personal skills like listening, dialogue, and working within a team. They also described how they had managed through the activities to explore individual differences among their own children, which ultimately called for different approaches in attending to their developmental growth.

Impressions of the workshops on women:

N: "We and our children feel frightened as a result of being continuously exposed to violations by Israeli soldiers and settlers like detention, assault, and physical inspection, let alone the emotional and mental damage caused by the news over media channels. Therefore, workshops are important because they help us deal with our personal and family daily life pressures, and also increase awareness of new topics and issues such as different forms of violence, electronic violations, and communication with our children—which is of utmost importance."

A: "The suffering caused by the fact that settlements are built on the lands of our village Twaneh in addition to the permanent presence of soldiers and closures have greatly affected my mental health. I feel nervous, have nightmares, and constantly fear that my kids will suffer from school underachievement, loss of desire for learning, lack of concentration and forgetfulness. However, our participation in the workshops, as well as targeting our children at school are considered important because they help us reduce negative feelings, increase understanding of the important topics that affect our lives, and introduce new skills in order to face our challenges."

K: "Awareness workshops help us identify all kinds of violence in addition to the mechanisms to combat, overcome, and mitigate its psychological and social repercussions. This is crucial in attending to the violence to which our children are exposed, gaining new information on how to deal with our kid's problems and behaviors, and ultimately offering them the needed support and help to overcome these problems. Now I have become able to express my feelings and my thoughts during the debate and dialogue sessions that took place on personal, family, and community levels."

A: "The difficulties and pressures of life that I face both on community and family levels make me feel nervous and unable to control my temper. Attending the workshops on different topics like combating violence and participating in activities related to children's problems and community have raised my knowledge, developed my personality, and increased my self-confidence and self-control. Having the counseling educator as a close person whom we trust, learn from, and exchange experiences with is of great importance. This gives us the opportunity to talk about our own experiences and ourselves to explore new alternatives in facing crises and challenges."

Participants' recommendations:

- Women need to process and raise awareness about how to deal with psychological pressures that they and their children face on a daily basis, overcome anxiety or shyness, and control nervousness.
- Students can benefit from awareness workshops that emphasize the importance of education and motivate them toward high academic achievement.
- Women should be equipped with empowering skills and methods on a personal level.

- Children should be provided with individual and group psychosocial counseling necessary to deal with different situations and crises caused by the occupation and settlements. This recommendation was made by a school director whose school has no social counselor.

The following excerpts from articles that focus on one family offer a human face on the situation in Area C of the West Bank, with a specific focus on Susiya.

Amira Hass, "The High Court Allowed the Bulldozers to Return to Susiya," *Haaretz*, 2018

… On Sunday, Iman Nawaja, 38, was busy moving piles of clothes out of her home. Her "home" is sheets of cloth and tarpaulin stretched on a few iron arches. The rocks are the living room. Three days earlier, on February 1, the High Court of Justice gave the go-ahead to demolish the arched structure, because it had been built without a permit, after an interim order had already been issued forbidding the state from demolishing structures in the village. Nawaja wanted to save the clothes of her family-of-seven first. She arranged the mattresses and blankets in the structure's southern corner. Their turn to be saved will come later. The nearby storeroom will also be torn down, the justices had ruled. The kitchen—an ancient, sheet-covered structure—is not on the Civil Administration's current demolition list…. The villagers cannot count the times the Israeli bulldozers have demolished structures, caves, water cisterns and agricultural terraces. Despite that, they always returned to the site. It's also hard to remember all the High Court sessions that were held in their case. The Palestinians want an approved master plan for their village. The Civil Administration wants them to live near Yatta, an urban community south of Hebron. It's good for the women, the administration officials wrote once.…

Jihad Nawaja, a neighbor and relative, remembers that June 1991 day as if it were yesterday. It was a Friday, and he and Mohammad had driven a tractor delivering straw to Yatta, for storage. They prayed and returned together. Jihad hadn't even turned the tractor's ignition off when they heard shots. "I saw the settler shooting the sheep, like a cowboy in a Western," he says. He thinks about 10 of the sheep were already killed. The shepherds crowded together to protect the rest of the herd. Jihad didn't mention or didn't remember anyone hitting the settler on the head.[7]

Nasser Nawaja, "Israel, Don't Level My Village," *New York Times,* July 23, 2015

SUSIYA, West Bank—In 1948, as Israeli forces closed in on his village of Qaryatayn, my grandfather carried my father in his arms to Susiya, about five miles north, in the South Hebron Hills area.

"We will go back home soon," my grandfather told my father.

They did not. Qaryatayn was destroyed, along with about 400 other Palestinian villages that were razed between 1948 and the mid-1950s. My family rebuilt their lives in Susiya, across the 1949 armistice line in the West Bank.

In 1986, my family was expelled from our home once again—not because of war, but because the occupying Israeli authorities decided to create an archaeological and tourist site around the remains of an ancient synagogue in Susiya. (A structure next to the abandoned temple was used as a mosque from about the 10th century.) This time, it was my father who took me in his arms as the soldiers drew near.

"We will return soon," he said.

We did not. Without compensation, we were forced to rebuild Susiya nearby on what was left of our agricultural lands.

If, in the coming weeks, the Israeli government carries out demolition orders served on some 340 residents of Susiya, I will be forced to take my children in my arms as our home is destroyed and the village razed once again. I do not know if I will have the heart to tell them that we will soon go home; history has taught me that it may be a very long time until we are able to return.... [8]

Appendix 3: Letters to elected representatives in the United States

Some members of the annual HATD Study Tour, all of whom were American, wrote letters to elected representatives in the United States. Below is an example of one letter that some members wrote to Senator Dianne Feinstein, at that time minority co-chair of the Senate Select Committee on Intelligence and a strong supporter of the Bedouin village of Susiya.

Dear Senator Feinstein,

We, the undersigned, took a study tour to Israel/West Bank in April of this year sponsored by an organization called Healing Across the Divides. As part of this study tour, we visited Palestinian and Israeli grantees that Healing Across the Divides funds, including one that provides counseling services to the women in Susiya. We are writing to simply thank you for your letters, hearings, and other interventions you've made on behalf of the Palestinian people living in this village and surrounding villages. We encourage you to continue to provide input on this important issue affecting thousands of very marginalized Palestinians. In addition to this letter we would be pleased to meet with you or your staff in Washington to give an in-person briefing.

I, Norbert Goldfield, as founder and executive director of Healing Across the Divides, a twelve-year-old organization, would like to emphasize that, very unusually, we take no political positions on the Israeli-Palestinian conflict. We focus on providing grants and technical services to community groups seeking to improve health for all marginalized Israelis and Palestinians. We are enclosing our 2015 annual report as further background to the work that we do in Israel and the West Bank.

In visiting these villages, we can attest to all the challenging situations that these Palestinians face that you highlighted in your letters and that emerged from the testimony. In fact, the organization providing counseling services has asked us for additional technical support, and we've budgeted additional funds to fly a colleague from the University of Pennsylvania, one of the world's experts on post-traumatic stress disorder among women. She will be conducting three days of training with therapists from this and other organizations in August. Her challenge is that the trauma is not post; it is ongoing.

In summary, thanks again for your interest in this issue. As I am sure you are fully aware, your personal intervention has made a life-saving difference for the Palestinian people living in Susiya. I will also follow up and see if we can set up a meeting with you and/or your staff.

Norbert Goldfield, M.D.
Executive Director
Healing Across the Divides
Northampton, MA

Notes

1 Naksa Day *Wikipedia* Available at: https://en.wikipedia.org/wiki/Naksa_Day. Accessed: June 20, 2020.
2 Susya. *Wikipedia* Available at: https://en.wikipedia.org/wiki/Susya. Accessed: June 20, 2020.
3 Patel, Y. (2018) Decades-long battle continues, as Susiya braces for more Israeli demolitions *Middle East Eye*. https://www.middleeasteye.net/news/decades-long-battle-continues-susiya-braces-more-israeli-demolitions. Accessed: June 29, 2020.
4 Israeli settler attacks against Palestinians 'tripled' (2019) Available at: https://www.youtube.com/watch?v=cDiSO24eb0s Accessed: June 20, 2020.

  Harel, A. (2018) Israeli 'Jewish terror' incidents targeting Palestinians tripled in 2018. *Haaretz*. Available at: https://www.haaretz.com/israel-news/.premium-israeli-jewish-terror-incidents-targeting-palestinians-tripled-in-2018–1.6809367. Accessed: June 20, 2020.
5 Hass, A. (2018) Israel to demolish entire west bank Bedouin Village, ending year-long legal battle. *Haaretz*. Available at: https://www.haaretz.com/israel-news/.premium-israel-to-demolish-entire-west-bank-bedouin-village-1.6116488. Accessed: January 1, 2019.
6 Human Rights Watch. (2006) *A Question of Security: Violence Against Palestinian Women and Girls*. https://www.hrw.org/report/2006/11/06/question-security/violence-against-palestinian-women-and-girls. Accessed: January 1, 2019.
7 Hass, A. (2018) The high court allowed the bulldozers to return to Susiya. *Haaretz*. Available at: https://www.haaretz.com/middle-east-news/palestinians/.premium-the-high-court-allowed-the-bulldozers-to-return-to-susya-1.5805805. Accessed: June 20, 2020
8 Nawaja, N. (2015) Israel, don't level my village. *The New York Times*. Available at: https://www.nytimes.com/2015/07/23/opinion/israel-dont-level-my-village.html. Accessed: June 20, 2020.

Chapter 13

White Hill Farm

Desert farming, improving nutrition and communication between Israeli Jews and Bedouin in Southern Israel

Norbert Goldfield

In this chapter, I will outline an HATD grant focused on a joint farming initiative between Israeli Jews and Bedouin in Southern Israel. This intervention is interesting and potentially important from more than a scientific perspective since, beyond that, the political and organizational trials and tribulations of its implementation represent a microcosm of the challenges and possibilities in trying to "heal across the divides" in this part of the world. I will provide a historical introduction to the geographic setting. I will then describe the organizations involved, the HATD-funded initiative, its preliminary results, and possible future directions. Research literature on community-supported agriculture in the United States has demonstrated that this type of effort can improve health. For example, a recently concluded randomized clinical trial documented that "community-supported agriculture intervention resulted in clinically meaningful improvements in diet quality."[1] In addition, with all the ongoing tension in the past decade between Israeli Bedouin and Israeli Jews, the White Hill Farm (WHF) is one of only a handful of efforts to concretely promote engagement in Israel today between these two groups.[2]

Historical introduction

According to the 1947 United Nations partition plan, the town of Beersheva (population approximately 5,000 at the time) in the Negev desert, in Southern Israel, was to be part of a new Palestinian state. The new state of Israel, founded in 1948 after the Israeli army defeated the Arab forces, included Beersheva, which then numbered 5,360 Muslims, 200 Christians, and 10 others living in the town.[3] At that time, the entire Negev desert had 90,000 Bedouin and 3,000 Jews.[4]

Today, Beersheva is the largest city in the Negev with a current population of more than 210,000 people. The modern town of Yeroham, established in 1951, currently has a population of approximately 11,000 Jews, a mostly low-income population, with 30% of the town's budget spent on welfare.

The Bedouin are largely nomadic Arabs who live throughout much of the Middle East. Prior to the founding of Israel, the Negev's population consisted almost entirely of Bedouin. Rachmeh, the name of the Bedouin village adjacent to Yeroham, is the partner with Yeroham in the joint urban farming project described below. It currently has a population of about 1,500. Rachmeh, like many Bedouin villages, is "unrecognized," meaning it doesn't have the benefit of any government services or infrastructures, such as electricity and other modern amenities. The lack of recognition stems from an ongoing dispute between Bedouin and the Israeli government over land ownership in the Negev.[5] The Israeli government continues to try and force the Bedouin off their lands and into government-approved towns. This has led to frequent clashes.[6]

The organizations involved

Earth's Promise was established in 2007 as a grassroots environmental and social change organization, funded by those interested in supporting sustainability, reviving neglected spaces, and bringing nature close to home. HATD awarded it a grant in 2018 to establish an agricultural center in Yeroham and Rachmeh. Unfortunately, shortly after the participants from Yeroham and Rachmeh started the farm with substantial effort, all the plants they had bought for the project were stolen. While HATD would have stopped the project immediately, the town of Yeroham, and the local nonprofit Atid Bamidbar, which runs an incubator for Bedouin and Jewish initiatives and organizes projects that promote relations with Rachmeh, decided to step in. An allocation from the Ministry of Agriculture via the Yeroham municipality paid for new plantings, the municipality provided boulders to fence the farm, and the project resumed, though not without considerable difficulty.

Atid Bamidbar is the current administrator of the White Hill Farm initiative (WHF). WHF is one of nearly twenty projects in

Atid Bamidbar's incubator for Bedouin-Jewish initiatives, implemented together with the "Neighbors" grassroots citizens' group (*Mirkam Azori*) and Bedouin colleagues from Rachmeh.

Rachmeh Residents Committee is the elected representative of the Bedouin living in Rachmeh.

The joint Bedouin-Jewish initiative

Initially, Earth's Promise envisioned an Ecological Agriculture Center, including a desert food forest, family garden rows, a traditional herb garden, and olive trees for a mutual olive harvest. It also called for the creation of an educational program to teach kindergarten children, the teachers, and the children's parents how to access fresh food and how proper nutrition can improve overall health and well-being. After assuming responsibility for this initiative, Atid Bamidbar continued the activities of Earth's Promise. In addition, Atid Bamidbar has been organizing regular meetings of a Rachmeh-Yeroham Women's Group with Bedouin and Jewish women; with HATD technical assistance, the staff recruited local women doctors and health specialists to introduce health-related discussions in informal, intimate meetings. Separately, thanks to Atid Bamidbar enlisting its support, the Ministry of Health initiated and has been conducting regular Healthy Cooking workshops for Bedouin women.

With the transition to Atid Bamidbar, the overall goals became to:

1 Promote mutual acquaintance, positive, peaceful neighborly relations, and engagement between Jews and Bedouin.
2 Develop and deepen participants' connection to nature and to healthy lifestyles, including increased knowledge and hands-on experience of both.
3 Develop the White Hill Farm as a replicable model for other neighboring communities of Jews and Arabs elsewhere in Israel's Negev and beyond.

Specific objectives included the following:

1 Deepen and expand weekly activities with Bedouin and Jewish kindergartens at WHF, involving Jewish and Bedouin kindergartens

active on the same day and times, teaching about elements of a healthy lifestyle and reaching parents from both communities via their children.

2   Develop a cadre of Bedouin and Jewish future leaders of the Farm via a training course for men in sustainable Negev agriculture integrating Bedouin knowledge.

3   Promote health-centered activities with Jews and Bedouin participating together at the Farm, such as the Healthy Cooking workshops.

4   Provide additional opportunities to deepen mutual acquaintance between Jews and Bedouin via various activities (community/ holiday events, Yeroham-Rachmeh Women's Group meetings), with an emphasis on activities at the Farm.

5   Develop the Farm as a replicable model for neighboring communities of Jews and Arabs, including demonstrating the model to kindergarten supervisors and teachers (from the Neve Midbar Bedouin Regional Council and elsewhere), as well as to visitors from Israel and abroad.

6   Maintain and develop the physical infrastructures of the Farm (trees, bushes, plots for planting, pergola, irrigation, etc.) as the foundation for all the above.

7   Identify potential partners, Bedouin and Jewish, to ensure the Farm's sustainability into the future.

The initiative is measuring/will measure three outcomes:

a   Change in nutrition-related knowledge and behavior, for both the Israeli Jewish and the Israeli Bedouin participants.
b   Change in number of participants at the WHF.
c   Change in communication between the Israeli Jewish and Israeli Bedouin participants in this initiative.

Cultural context of this initiative

Ties between Jewish residents of Yeroham and Bedouin residents of Rachmeh have developed over the past five decades. They have expanded in amount and scope since the "Neighbors" (Mirkam Azori) citizens' group was founded by Yeroham residents in 2005, and since Atid Bamidbar opened its incubator for Bedouin-Jewish initiatives in 2017.

One of the expressions of the augmented relationship, the fruit of joint Jewish and Bedouin efforts, is the opening of a Ministry of Education kindergarten in Rachmeh (now increased to three kindergartens) and the imminent opening of the Rachmeh Elementary School, scheduled for September 1, 2020. Mutual social visits, help with bureaucracy, Yeroham pupils visiting Rachmeh residents, Hebrew tutoring of Rachmeh residents, the Ajram Bedouin's women sewing initiative, joining forces for intensive work in tourism activities (especially via Atid Bamidbar, 200 groups per year who visited Rachmeh in 2019)—these are all other expressions of the ongoing and positive relationships between Yeroham's leadership and residents and Rachmeh's leadership and residents.

An important part of Atid Bamidbar's incubator is the "Good Neighbors Network in the Negev," a platform for joint activities between adjacent Jewish and Bedouin localities, mostly unrecognized villages. Here Bedouin and Jewish social activists work together to promote good neighborly relations and overcome ignorance, alienation, and hostility, deepen mutual acquaintance, and work together on various activities, projects, and events, including influencing policy makers to improve the situation in Bedouin settlements in the Negev.

It is against this background that Atid Bamidbar took over responsibility for the management and development of the White Hill Farm in June 2018, as a venue for mutual encounter, deepening acquaintance, and connecting to healthy lifestyles and to nature among both Rachmeh and Yeroham residents. Given the critical importance of promoting health in both poor communities, the WHF project has led Atid Bamidbar to growing involvement in this field. WHF leaders enlisted the partnership of the Ministry of Health to promote Healthy Cooking workshops, a national pilot for the Ministry, among Bedouin women in the unrecognized villages. This Ministry is also funding additional activities in both localities—soccer for Rachmeh youth, and nutrition workshops for Jewish kindergarten pupils, teachers, and parents in Yeroham.

At the same time, WHF leaders faced numerous challenges in implementing the initiative that they took over from Earth's Promise.

WHF leaders did not anticipate, for example, the Bedouin drivers' strikes that made it impossible to bring Rachmeh children to the Farm for encounters with the Jewish children during several months in 2019 and early 2020. That is why in 2020 the WHF has arranged to pay for 30 days of transportation to the farm for Bedouin children, with an eye to holding four to six mutual activities with Jewish children in four Jewish and three Bedouin kindergartens.

Following the principle of egalitarian representation, in the sustainable agriculture course funded in part by the Israel Lands Authority's Open Lands Fund, the WHF involves 5 Bedouin and 5 Jews. The steering committee for the project includes Bedouin and Jewish leaders equally. The joint Women's Group is usually half Bedouin women and half Jewish women at each session (which usually numbers around 15–20 from each locality). But not all the projects can be exactly fifty-fifty. The joint Iftar (a Muslim holiday) that WHF organized in May 2019 drew more or less equal numbers of Jews and Bedouin, but no Bedouin women; the same is true for the communal events, except for Hanukkah, when WHF leaders paid the Bedouin women to lead the crafts workshops. WHF leaders make many efforts to incorporate Bedouin in all activities on an equal basis, but cultural and social constraints in Rachmeh work against this goal.

Yeroham has been especially active during the COVID-19 crisis on behalf of the unrecognized village of Rachmeh. Throughout March, April, and May 2020, the Mayor of Yeroham and concerned Yeroham citizen colleagues worked in concert with Bedouin in Rachmeh to stop the distribution of demolition orders and attempts to dig up sown wheat fields. A letter was sent by the Good Neighbors Network members to government Ministries and the Prime Minister, which resulted in a temporary respite and an unusual public statement from the head of the Bedouin Settlement Authority against digging up sown wheat fields and demolition orders during the crisis. However, the demolition orders have since been renewed. The work, including ongoing contact with Bedouin, documentation, contact with the authorities, and reaching out to media, continues to this day to protect the unrecognized village of Rachmeh. Moreover, during the first months of the COVID-19 crisis, in cooperation with Yeroham's mayor and the Home Front Command, the Ministries of Health, Labor, Social Affairs and Social Services, and Justice, WHF staff played a critical role in distributing food packages and games to Rachmeh families, as well as essential information in Arabic about the virus, hygiene, keeping safe, and civil rights.

Summary of preliminary findings

- **Joint Jewish–Bedouin Women's Group:** This joint group convenes every few weeks. Most of the women (89% Jews, 78% Bedouin) have attended encounters for more than a year. Jewish women felt that the encounters strengthened ties and even encouraged friendships to develop with the Bedouin women. Some of the Rachmeh women noted that the encounters provide them with a rare opportunity to get out of the house and be in the company of other women. Half of the Rachmeh women said that they were positively surprised by the encounters and continue to come in order to learn about and teach the customs of the two communities. One of the Bedouin women disclosed that she began to come to the encounters because of the nourishing meals for her and her children but stayed and came again and again because she found it of great social interest. The encounters also led to changing perceptions of the other. Most of the women in both communities reported that the encounters altered their perceptions of the women from the other community as they learned more about them. In addition, the Bedouin women noted an increased desire to learn Hebrew, a sense of belonging to both communities (thanks to visiting each other's homes), more knowledge of Jewish customs, and an increased acceptance of divergent opinions.
- **Women's Cooking Workshops:** Ministry of Health staff facilitated Healthy Cooking workshops with Bedouin women from Rachmeh, at the Farm and at women's homes. The Ministry covered most of the cost of the workshops; Atid Bamidbar purchased raw materials and equipment as needed. WHF held six such workshops during 2019. In addition, some of the women who participated in the workshops, and other women from Rachmeh, came to the Farm and/or were exposed by the Rachmeh kindergarten teacher to the principles of healthy eating via their children in the kindergarten who visited the Farm on a regular basis. Also, some of the same women, and additional women from Rachmeh,

participated in meetings of the Rachmeh-Yeroham Women's Group, where health issues, including healthy nutrition, were discussed informally in an intimate atmosphere.

- **Kindergarten Nutrition Program:** At the Farm, the children eat only healthy food that they pick fresh or bring. The Healthy Cooking workshops continue with health-oriented encounters of the Women's Group. They integrate health-related workshops in communal events. The impact of the cooking workshops is being measured using a pre- and post-initiative design and a validated nutrition questionnaire in Hebrew and Arabic. Thus far, from an anecdotal perspective, it can be seen that being at the Farm has had positive effects on the kindergarten children from both communities, leading to healthier diets and increased physical activity, motoric skills, self-confidence, and curiosity about nature. The sample size is too small for firm conclusions.

Discussion

WHF represents another example of the type of high-risk grant-making decisions that HATD has undertaken since its founding in 2004. While this is a challenging initiative and may easily fail (we will not know until at least the end of 2021), the reward potential is very high. Imagine the impact of such a joint farming initiative between Israeli Jews and Israeli Bedouin if replicated throughout the Negev. Imagine the impact of such an endeavor on improved nutrition and improved communication between these two groups.

Challenging as it is, this very type of high-risk initiative goes to the heart of what Healing Across the Divides is trying to accomplish. Even if it fails, all parties—Israeli Jews, Israeli Bedouin, and all HATD grantees—will learn from the failure. But we continue to be hopeful that the White Hill Farm will succeed in improving nutrition and communication between two groups throughout the Negev who have historically had a fraught relationship.

Notes

1 Berkowitz, SA., O'Neill, J., Sayer, E., et al. (2019) Health center-based community-supported agriculture: An RCT. *Am J Prev Med.* 57 (6 Suppl 1), pp: S55–S64.

2 Al-Said, H, Braun-Lewensohn, O., Sagy, S. (2018) Sense of coherence, hope, and home demolition are differentially associated with anger and anxiety among Bedouin Arab adolescents in recognized and unrecognized villages. *Anxiety Stress Coping.* 31(4), pp: 475–485.

   Eglash, R. (2016) After decades of service, some Bedouins aren't sure about joining the Israeli army. *Washington Post* Available at https://www.washingtonpost.com/world/middle_east/somebedouins-arent-sure-about-serving-israel-army/2016/05/28/f84e2db6-1249-11e6-a9b5-bf703a5a7191_story.html. Accessed: June 14, 2020.

3 Beersheva *Wikipedia* Available at: https://en.wikipedia.org/wiki/Beersheba Accessed: June 13, 2020 Beersheva Municipality. Demographic Data Available at https://www.beer-sheva.muni.il/Eng/About/Pages/Figures.aspx Accessed: June 13, 2020.

4 Suwaed, MW. (2015). Bedouin-Jewish relations in the Negev 1943–1948. *Middle Eastern Studies* 51 (5), pp: 767–788.

5 Abu-Saad, K. (2014) State-directed 'development' as a tool for dispossessing the Indigenous Palestinian Bedouin-Arabs in the Naqab in: Turner M Shweiki O *Decolonizing Palestinian political economy: de-development and beyond.* London: Palgrave Macmillan, pp: 138–157.

6 Ziv, O. (2020) Israel steps up campaign against Bedouin village it demolished 173 times *972 Magazine.* (Journal online) January 28, 2020. Available at: https://www.972mag.com/al-araqib-demolished-bedouin/. Accessed: March 22, 2020.

   Okbi, Y. (2019) Bedouins forced to destroy their own homes in the Negev, *The Jerusalem Post.* Available at: https://www.jpost.com/Israel-News/Bedouins-forced-to-destroy-their-own-homes-in-the-Negev-594362. Accessed: June 13, 2020.

Chapter 14

Strengthening women leaders since Healing Across the Divides was founded in 2004

Christine Seibold

Introduction

The long-standing Israeli-Palestinian conflict has had a significant economic, social, religious, emotional, and physical impact on Israelis and Palestinians. This chapter will provide a summary of recent research work that I conducted in partial fulfillment of my graduate degree,[1] which sought to answer the following questions: Does attempting to improve health for people living in Israel and Occupied Palestinian Territory (OPT) through Healing Across the Divides' (HATD) engagement in the community facilitate peace building? Does offering opportunities for mutual engagement to the two groups through health break down tension and barriers? Can cooperation between program participants in Israel and OPT change the attitudes of citizens who suffer from the Israeli-Palestinian conflict? How, if at all, does HATD funding and, more importantly, the technical/organizational engagement of HATD impact grantee leadership?

I hypothesized that foundations such as Healing Across the Divides can help improve health, break down relational borders between Israelis and Palestinians, and facilitate peace building between them. I tested this by creating surveys and reviewing those completed and submitted by grantees, as well as conducting interviews with female leaders of several HATD-funded organizations. I also hypothesized that HATD's active engagement with its grantees would result in changes in the attitudes and behavior of the (mostly female) leadership of HATD grantees.

This chapter is divided into several sections. Under "Methods," I describe the tools I used for this research. I then describe the results of this research, except for the section of HATD's impact on grantee leadership. I conclude with the results of interviews with female leaders of HATD grantees. For this chapter, I interviewed six women between December 2019 and February 2020. These women work in leadership positions in HATD grantee organizations. In brief, all six of them agreed that Healing Across the Divides has had a profound impact on their ability to lead, as well as to improve the organizations in which they work.

Method

I collected four types of data. The main source of data was obtained from questionnaires filled out by those who work and participate in programs with HATD. Second, I interviewed the director, staff, and board members of HATD. For a third type of data, I attended, observing and taking notes, a joint meeting of all Israeli and Palestinian HATD grantees willing to meet that was held in East Jerusalem on December 5, 2017. Finally, I held face-to-face meetings in December 2019 with and/or interviewed via the Internet from December 2019 through February 2020 several women leaders of the organizations funded by Healing Across the Divides. I guaranteed all grantee participants that all personal judgments of HATD that might identify the respondent were to be masked; thus, no one, including the executive director (Norbert Goldfield), could identify the respondents.

I received 54 completed questionnaires and interviewed six leaders in all. However, many staff members of the community-based organizations and participants refused to complete my research questionnaires because of some of the political questions related to the conflict, and/or they did not trust the origin of the questionnaire. I supported my findings with a literature review of the field of peace building through health.

Overall results

My research found that from a qualitative perspective, the overall health of the participants that HATD serves is improving. I also found that positive communication, interaction, and an increase in trust, elements necessary for breaking down relational borders and moving toward peace, are present to some degree. HATD is moving in the right direction by facilitating joint meetings, cross-communication, and the sharing of resources between Israeli and Palestinian staff. These actions are essential to forming trusting relationships and understanding one another, ingredients that lead toward peace. The following three subsections discuss the impact of HATD-funded programs on community health, the breaking down of relational borders, and facilitating peace-building activities.

Results: Improve public health

Fifty percent of Palestinian participants in HATD grantee programs who responded agreed that their HATD program improved their health and/or their families' health. While the Israeli participants had no opinion, most had refused to complete the questionnaire. Of the 20 Palestinian program staff members who completed the questionnaire, 65% agreed that the health of the groups that they work with had improved. In addition, both Israeli staff and Palestinian staff who live in Israel (4 total) said they agreed and strongly agreed that the health had improved in the groups that they serve. One of the staff, for example, commented that hundreds of women are now more aware of the risks of obesity, and that participants increased their awareness about unhealthy behaviors such as smoking, drinking alcohol, and the negative effects on the body.

Results: Break down relational borders between Israelis and Palestinians

Fifty percent of Palestinian participants (20 total) said that by participating in the HATD program, they had the potential to learn and understand different viewpoints of Israelis and to increase overall trust between Israelis and Palestinians living in the Occupied Palestinian Territory (OPT). Thirty-five percent of the Palestinian participants agreed that participating in the HATD program has the potential to facilitate positive communication or interaction between Israelis and Palestinians through new programs in the future, which would be a step toward working together and breaking down relational borders.

Fifty-five percent of Palestinian staff in the OPT, Israeli Jewish staff, Palestinian staff in Israel, board members, and both HATD representatives agreed or strongly agreed that working with HATD has helped them to learn and understand different viewpoints of Palestinians and Israeli Jews. Fifty-five percent of Palestinian staff said they have witnessed a positive change in the attitudes of Palestinians toward Israelis and Palestinians living in Israel. One of the Israeli staff and one of the Palestinian staff in Israel also agreed. The two representatives both agreed that working with HATD programs has positively influenced their own views and attitudes toward Israelis and Palestinians.

Positive communication, interaction, and increased trust are elements needed for breaking down relational borders and moving toward peace. A majority agreed that HATD can facilitate, or already has facilitated, an increase in positive relations between the groups in Israel and the OPT, as well as understanding others' views. One of the staff members suggested organizing community dialogues for people to share their stories to build empathy. A second employee agreed that HATD should persist in its efforts to facilitate networking between the staff so that they could continue learning about one another.

Results: Facilitate peace building
between Israelis and Palestinians

Only 35% of Palestinian participants agreed that involvement in the HATD program has the potential to provide a foundation for Israelis and Palestinians living in the OPT to break down barriers and begin building peace. Sixty percent of the Palestinian staff in the OPT and 100% of the board members thought the HATD initiatives have the potential to provide a foundation for Israelis and Palestinians to break down barriers and begin building peace.

Some of the HATD board members commented that building peace in the region at this time seems possible only through working with communities from the bottom up. They thought that not focusing on politics and peace building but continuing to focus on improving the health of the participants should remain at the core of HATD's mission. They were in agreement that continuing to facilitate joint workshops in a neutral area in order to exchange experiences and knowledge is important.

Results: How HATD has affected women's leadership (interviews)

The first woman I interviewed has been with her non-governmental organization (NGO) for nineteen years. She manages workers, counselors, hospitals, and municipalities. She also teams up with other NGOs. She handles new partnerships with the local government and is in charge of operating programs. She works with the central government and the Ministry of Health to help create a national plan of action.

She stated that having HATD's assistance has given her the foundation to serve her clients in impactful ways. She has been working with volunteers for many years. The project with HATD has taught her how to function more effectively, to define goals and to be more visible in the community, which in turn has led to the success of the program. With HATD's backing, she has felt truly supported and engaged, which has made it possible for her to deal with challenges in positive ways.

The second woman I interviewed has been working in her NGO for twenty-five years. She frequently engages with the Ministry of Health and other directors of ministries, businesses, and commercial companies to build the NGO and bring knowledge about the target audience to the community. She also deals with the marketing and digital side of the organization.

She says that HATD has been an amazing partnership. It was the first time she was able to learn how to work with an organization that pulls its weight in a project and is a true teammate. She had dealt with funders previously, but the experience was not the same. HATD has taught her new ways of working with a donor and how to cooperate to solve problems. The leadership of HATD has kept their word in what they promised to help with since the beginning. She also agrees that she learned new leadership skills while partnering with HATD.

The third woman I interviewed has been directing her NGO for eighteen years. Over this period, she has served as a liaison to the current manager, has been responsible for training, developing projects and ideas, mobilizing resources, and implementing, evaluating, and submitting reports. She also has been in charge of expanding membership in the organization and working with local, national, and international communities and organizations.

HATD has been supporting her organization for the past three years. There is no doubt that its involvement has had an impact on her as a leader in the organization, mainly in strengthening cooperation tools and assessment tools, as well as expanding the membership/leadership network within the organization. In addition, it has served as a reference tool for the organization and a link to the community.

The fourth woman I interviewed has worked briefly for her organization as Director of the HATD project. The project educates and implements activities for men, women, and families with a chronic illness. Before coming to the organization, she was a volunteer for years with a women's center in a village where she lives. She has a university degree; however, she worked at home for years raising her children. Now that she is employed outside the home, she feels more empowered and that it is important to take care of herself. Until very recently this organization was made up of only men. The fact that a woman is now leading it demonstrates her strength as a leader.

The fifth woman that I interviewed is a coordinator in the organization that oversees an HATD-funded initiative. She explained that she married young and didn't finish school. She later went back and graduated from high school and college and then became a social worker. She volunteered at a camp in her village and worked as a volunteer in a variety of institutions. Now she is a teacher of groups of women. She thinks that feeling proud as a mother and woman while employed is important and sets an example for other Palestinian women. Both leaders from the chronic disease program encourage other women to participate in activities, meetings, exercise, awareness, and camps for children.

Because of the support that HATD has given to the NGO, both of these women have more responsibilities than when they previously worked as volunteers. In the beginning, they said, it was good to be a volunteer, but now they feel empowered because they are earning their own salary and making decisions within the organization. One of the biggest wins for them as women leaders was the reaction of men on the board; after witnessing their success in this project, they now look to them for advice and opinions. The women were even invited to join the board, which, as employees of the organization, they cannot do. However, they are proud to be leading the way and setting an example for women to come.

The sixth woman that I interviewed, with fifteen years' experience in her organization, works in the areas of training, educating, teaching at universities, and as a consultant to organizations. As a consultant for psychosocial support for women and children, she strives for the prevention and empowering awareness of women's abuse in the OPT. Besides holding workshops for men, women, and mothers and overseeing many volunteers, she engages with other women's associations and advocates for family law protection, for the change and implementation of the law to benefit women.

The all-male advisory board of her organization invites her to their meetings. They seek her out and look to her for advice because they believe in her and her decisions and planning. This woman consults with an organization concerned with violence against women in the OPT. Her leadership position has enabled her to communicate the needs of abused women at the shelter and to transfer ideas about how to deal with them to the board.

I personally left all of these interviews feeling empowered by these women, impressed by the leadership positions that they achieved and have held over the last twenty years. It is clear that HATD has made sustained efforts to increase the leadership skills of these women, helping them to acquire the skills to face adversity in a positive way so that they and their organizations can be successful. All six women I interviewed expressed gratitude for HATD's guidance in learning leadership skills, encouraging their growth as individuals and in their organizational roles.

Leading from within: participants who have become leaders

Through the work with Healing Across the Divides, various people involved with HATD-funded groups have developed and grown into leaders in their organizations. Many of them started out as participants and then became passionate about the work and took on a leadership role. Some of the directors themselves have also grown into different leadership roles throughout the years.

The program that recruited grandmothers to take charge of a home-safety intervention (see chapter 6) has enabled the volunteer grandmothers to become leaders in their community. Paraphrasing one of these volunteer grandmother leaders I interviewed: "The community now looks to the grandmothers as VIP representatives in their own society. In the past, women have not been recognized for their roles. However, when the grandmothers go on the streets and the people are working together as a community, they stay healthier. It is beautiful to see grandmothers who were shy and low in social 'status' now become leaders. The mayor of the community and people in the streets now look to them as leaders, which is a dramatic change and is due to the program."

The leader of the organization that runs workshops and trainings for people with diabetes noted that its project has given visibility to a lot of people. In the beginning, the participants of the project were shy and afraid to express their opinions. The program helped them gain confidence and become more communicative. Furthermore, many participants made it possible for family members to realize that they had diabetes as they all learned more about the disease, which has led to faster and more effective treatment for these family members.

The leader of the organization that educates and assists women who are victims of domestic violence uses her experience to teach students in college how to be leaders in domestic abuse treatment. These women teach other women in the organization how to spread the word about these difficult issues and where they can get help. This, in turn, has had positive effects when the students went out in the field seeking employment, as such volunteer, hands-on experiences gave them credibility on their résumés. Half of the people from the first year of the program were able to get a job in this field. Through the program, they work in the areas of public speaking, confidence, and training others, which in turn, creates new leaders in society.

In addition, the organization's manager was originally one of the participants in the HATD-funded initiative. Teams of women participants are in charge of the volunteer hotline program. Her involvement with this program led to her promotion as manager. Other women who participated in the hotline/aid center program later took part in the local behavioral network training project. Today they have leadership roles and work throughout different areas of the OPT.

Leading together with other organizations

All of the women who were interviewed noted that partnering with Healing Across the Divides has had a significant, positive impact on relationship building between the community organizations that they support and other organizations, such as the Ministry of Health and other ministries. The HATD grantees and some ministries have worked together toward common goals and have increased their organizational capacity in marketing and digital advertising. By joining forces with others, they have improved their strategic work values, goal setting, and effective communication. Other HATD grantees have, as a consequence of HATD encouragement and assistance, connected with hospitals or with the Ministry of Education to implement educational programs in schools and universities.

HATD also helped considerably with a project that led to the creation of a local leadership network. The network represented seven localities that promoted programmatic cooperation between welfare, health, and community institutions within the towns. None of the programs would have been developed had the project not been supported and nurtured. During the project, the HATD meetings with the foundation's grantees produced and promoted joint efforts among the various organizations.

One of the women interviewed concluded by saying that making a change and working with other organizations is a marathon, not a sprint. One has to have a lot of patience, especially when dealing with organizations that have different goals and systems. She commented that every step you take is toward the top of the mountain. And if you continue taking step by step, you will reach the goal.

Lessons from being a leader

These six women who were interviewed as leaders have gained many lessons from their work in their organizations and from support and partnering with Healing Across the Divides. One woman said that she has learned that the greatest asset to an organization is its people. And when a group of people wants to reach the stars and the moon, they will do it even though they will encounter many challenges. She has come to believe in people and has seen others who are aligned with the organization's goals do great things.

A second woman shared that she learned how important it is to have partnerships with others that have a common goal. Communication and transparency are key to being successful because communication leads to trust. Furthermore, she now feels that engaging with other people through transparency will bring you a long way toward trust. She points to the immense value of connecting with members of the community and the significance of knowing how to speak the language of your audience, and she has come to understand the importance of creating local leadership that will be a pillar between the organization and its community in the future.

Others related that they have experienced many difficulties and problems arising from the customs of the society in which they work, such as keeping women safe, or even something as "simple as" having a place for women to exercise where they feel comfortable. Yet they have learned how to take problems and challenges and, bringing off positive change from negative situations, found solutions and created opportunities for communities to succeed. Some women recounted that they acquired critical skills as leaders while participating in various trainings, where they learned about discrimination against women, combating obesity and depression, and women and self-esteem.

Finally, I spoke with a woman who, just a few years ago, did not have the same rights that she now has. Today, she is a decision maker and a successful person in her society. She makes changes in her community and her organization. From her experience in being supported by HATD, she personally became more open-minded and can now solve issues related to her family. As a woman, she does not need to stay at home. She has become strong and empowered enough to decide what she wants as a woman and as a leader and to carry it out. She no longer feels limited and will continue to keep learning and growing.

The Israeli-Palestinian conflict and leadership

When asked how their role as a leader has been challenged or affected because of the political situation between Israel and the OPT, there was little or no response.

One woman stated that there has been no impact related to the programs they are running. She mentioned there was one occasion that Palestinians from the Occupied Palestinian Territory (OPT) were planning to work with the grandmother project in Israel (see chapter 6). They had one meeting with some people from the organization sponsoring the grandmother's project, but it did not become a joint Israeli-Palestinian initiative because the Palestinian grantee did not want to work with them. The Israeli army also would not give permits to people from the OPT to come to Israel for meetings. She said they try not to mix politics and work.

Another woman asserted that no problems related to the conflict have affected her organization. Another stated that it has not had an effect on her as a leader, but the checkpoints and soldiers have caused meetings to be postponed or moved. Finally, the last woman commented that the political situation undoubtedly has had an effect on her work in the organization in ways she did not want to expand on, but the political situation has never stopped her from doing her job or being a leader.

From an outsider's perspective, I have no doubt that the situation affects these leaders both personally and professionally on a regular basis; however, they do not want to talk about it. It seems that the current way of life in both Israel and the OPT has become "normal" to them. Because of that, perhaps they no longer even notice the ways they are affected. I myself saw effects with my own eyes when I attended the joint meeting in December 2017. Some people were not able to attend because they could not get permission to cross from the OPT to East Jerusalem (claimed by both Israel and the OPT but annexed by Israel) where the meeting was held. One woman had to hide the fact that she was at a meeting with "the other side" from her husband or he would not have allowed her to attend, as he is not supportive of such meetings. One man had to leave the meeting early, because some soldiers were destroying his neighbor's home and he was worried about his children's safety.

Unfortunately, this is their truth right now and has been for years. It is clear that both sides try to do what they can within the situation and live each day to the best of their ability. On a positive note, it is good to see that no one who was interviewed feels that the political situation has affected them as individual leaders.

Limitations of this work

A significant limitation in my research was that much of the literature is biased due to strong opinions about the ongoing conflict. The Israeli-Palestinian conflict leaves no room for middle ground; many feel very passionate and "right" about their theories and opinions around the history, current problems, and solutions to the conflict. A second limitation is that a significant percentage of both populations have "tuned out" the conflict and are simply trying to live their lives in whichever way they can. Often, because of fear, they are not interested in engaging with other groups outside their own immediate community. This led many to not answer either specific questions and/or entire questionnaires.

A third limitation was the difficulty in choosing appropriate language when describing the Israeli-Palestinian conflict. Since many Palestinians will not acknowledge the State of Israel and many Israelis do not acknowledge the possibility of a Palestinian state, it can be difficult when explaining the conflict or referencing it to one side or the other. In addition, many people on both sides of the issue find the problems so personally devastating that they felt some questions concerning the issue were invasive, and therefore were hesitant to respond to the questionnaires.

Conclusion

My research indicates that HATD-funded initiatives are improving the health of their Israeli and Palestinian participants and have caused a positive change in attitudes toward one another. However, responses to the questionnaires and interviews indicated that HATD does not directly contribute to peace building in the Israeli-Palestinian conflict. Yet, as a final summing up, my research showed that HATD initiatives have the potential to provide a foundation for Israelis and

Palestinians to break down barriers and begin building peace in the future. It also shows that it has strengthened the NGOs that HATD funds and, in some cases, helped to strengthen their leaders. HATD has furnished these leaders with valuable tools, resources, and support that enable them to grow and flourish, personally, as individual leaders within their organizations, and throughout their community.

Note

1 Seibold, C. (2018). *Peace building between Israel – Palestine: Eliminating borders through public health initiatives.* Masters Thesis. Harvard University, Cambridge, MA.

Part III

Is peace building through health possible in a setting of the Israeli-Palestinian conflict? Past, present, future

Can health professionals effectively engage in "healing across the divides" in a setting of ongoing conflict?

Norbert Goldfield

Introduction

Peace Building through Health (PtH) should be in decline. What with increasing attacks on health professionals, only made worse by the COVID-19 pandemic,[1] and significant challenges to humanitarian aid in general over the past two decades,[2] one would expect that fewer health professionals would be willing to put themselves in harm's way. And with more refugees in the world today than at any time since World War II, it would not be surprising if fewer health professionals proved willing to persist in a practice akin to banging their heads against a brick wall. But the reality is that health professionals will continue to respond to a moral calling to do this work even if some consider it quixotic or useless, let alone unnecessarily dangerous. For those of us health professionals who will at least try to mitigate the impact of conflicts and the humanitarian crises that emerge from them, the aim of this chapter is to outline recent challenges and opportunities in the PtH field, with a specific focus on the Israeli-Palestinian conflict.

I begin this chapter with challenges to humanitarian action, surely a bedrock feature of PtH. Over the past two decades, David Rieff, in particular, has eloquently provided us with a trenchant critique of this field.[3] Most recently, Doctors without Borders/Médecins sans Frontières has taken up the subject with an online set of commentaries on politics and humanitarianism.[4] I will tie together aspects of humanitarianism with salient features of PtH.

Next, I turn to the Israeli-Palestinian conflict. Only a few organizations, most notably Physicians for Human Rights (PHR)-Israel, have continuously and courageously worked with both Israelis and

Palestinians. I will comment on how PHR-Israel has internalized the Doctors without Borders manifesto published in 2019: "The act of providing humanitarian aid is deeply political. It is not an act of partisan politics but an act of resistance against a status quo in which people are prevented from accessing the basic means of survival, such as healthcare."[5]

Partly in response to the Oslo Accords signed in 1993 between Israel and the Palestine Liberation Organization (which became the Palestinian Authority), a small group of Israeli and Palestinian health professionals, under the auspices and leadership of local directors of the World Health Organization, jointly published the magazine *Bridges*. This chapter will analyze several of the articles from this magazine. The *Lancet*, one of the most important medical journals in the world, has been and continues to be engaged substantively with Israeli and Palestinian health professionals. This chapter will summarize the many controversies surrounding The *Lancet*'s ongoing engagement and its relationship to PtH.

While always present to a degree, relentless attacks (physical and verbal) against health professionals constitute a further relatively new challenge to PtH. These include, specifically, Israeli attacks on Palestinian health professionals. The next chapter deals with this topic. Finally, from 2010 to 2020, a number of journals, particularly *Medicine, Conflict and Survival*, have published several articles setting out new ways of looking at the role of PtH. These articles will be analyzed in this chapter with particular reference to the Israeli-Palestinian conflict. With these perspectives and information as background, I then conclude this chapter with a discussion of the political choices that HATD has made since its founding in 2004 in its effort to incorporate PtH within its mission.

Humanitarianism and its ties with PTH

David Rieff has highlighted in recent writings the challenges that attend humanitarianism and, by implication at least, aspects of PtH. "Humanitarianism was never the appropriate response to the boundless sufferings of the poor world.... But whether or not that bitter lesson has sunk in, and, more to the point, what the implications of this Promethean knowledge are for humanitarianism, is another matter."[6]

Or, as Roy Williams, the former director of the International Rescue Committee (IRC), puts it, "humanitarian organizations are not capable of dealing with the crises we see around us. There are no humanitarian solutions to humanitarian problems."[7] If organizations are to do more than place "Band-Aids over malignant tumors,"[8] PtH organizations involved in this type of action must face the limitations of political neutrality and, in fact, become more political.

At the same time, since the late twentieth century, a significant number of world leaders have encouraged just the opposite perspective—a "responsibility to protect" vulnerable populations at immediate risk from authoritarian regimes (such as the Rohingya in Myanmar). "What has gradually been emerging is a parallel transition from a culture of sovereign impunity to a culture of national and international accountability."[9] Unfortunately, the responsibility to protect movement, despite numerous publications and the political push of senior statesmen such as Kofi Annan and Jimmy Carter, has never gotten off the ground. Today, vulnerable populations have largely been abandoned, leading to the worst refugee crisis since World War II.[10]

This already difficult situation has become all the more complex as countries are increasingly using funds committed to humanitarian relief as mere extensions of foreign policy goals. Thus, for example, in a recently released call for proposals concerning cultural programs for Israel, the US Agency for International Development (USAID) explicitly states in its funding criteria that the program will be more highly rated if it "increases public understanding of the U.S.-Israel security partnership."[11] According to Andrew Natsios, the former director of the USAID,

> Foreign assistance is an important tool ... to further America's interests. In fact, it is sometimes the most appropriate tool when diplomacy is not enough or military force imprudent. Foreign assistance implements peace agreements arranged by diplomats and often enforced by the military; it supports peacekeeping efforts ... helps nations prepare for participation in the global economic system and become better markets for U.S. exports.[12]

What are the different approaches to PtH, with a focus on the situation confronting Israelis and Palestinians, that could thread this seemingly impossible needle? The next sections highlight developments in PtH since the late 1990s in the context of the Israeli-Palestinian conflict.

Israeli and Palestinian PTH organizational engagement from the 1990s to the present

The signing of the Oslo Accords in 1993 witnessed the significant funding of joint Israeli-Palestinian health care initiatives. Between 1994 and 1998, at a time of hope for a positive outcome for the Israeli-Palestinian conflict, analysis, as summarized by Barnea and colleagues, of 148 Israeli-Palestinian health initiatives by primary type of activity revealed that most of the projects were in the areas of training (46%), followed by research (23%) and service development (14%).[13] Three smaller areas covered conferences, seminars, dialogues, and youth activities (7%), service provision (5%), and policy planning (5%). Nine projects from the late 1990s provided specific examples of health-related outcomes, including:

- Training of health personnel (specialist training of 23 Palestinian physicians; accredited training in family medicine for 4 Palestinian physicians; training of 380 teachers as health educators).
- Development of infrastructure, specifically, contributing to the establishment of the Health Promotion and Education Directorate in the Palestinian Ministry of Health; establishment of a state-of-the-art laboratory at a Palestinian university.
- Direct provision of service to more than 20,000 Palestinians in rural areas and 80,000 students.
- Generation of data, to assist policy planning and development of intervention programs for both the Palestinian Authority and Israel in the fields of adolescent health behaviors, leishmaniasis, and beta-thalassemia (the latter two diseases are particularly endemic among Palestinians).

Many of these initiatives between 1994 and 1998 could be viewed as one-sided in the sense that Israelis typically assumed a leadership role and Palestinians from the Occupied Palestinian Territory (OPT) assumed the role of "student"—from an organizational and/or a technical point of view. Nonetheless, these initiatives led to Israeli-Palestinian communication and, in fact, the two sides working together. The vast majority of these joint efforts ceased after the beginning of the second intifada in 2000. One organization that has continued engagement between Israelis and Palestinians around health issues, albeit in a very modest manner, is the Shimon Peres Center for Peace. This organization has concentrated on the treatment of Palestinian children in Israeli hospitals and the training of Palestinian health professionals. Beginning in 2003 and through 2019, the Peres Center has funded, primarily with grants from the European Union, the treatment of 12,500 Palestinian children with, for example, congenital cardiac conditions from the OPT in Israeli hospitals and the training, as of 2019, of 250 Palestinian health professionals in Israeli institutions.[14]

The most active organization, Israeli or Palestinian, engaged with many PtH activities from its beginning in 1988 up to the first intifada, throughout the second intifada, and to the present, is Physicians for Human Rights-Israel.[15] This organization has engaged in virtually all aspects of PtH as described in Chapter 1. With respect to its work with Palestinians in the OPT, PHR-Israel "works to protect Palestinians' right to health. Appeals of patients & medical personnel reveal barriers to health posed by the occupation's military & civilian arms, and allow us to fight both specific violations & the oppressive policy itself."[16] In order to deliver direct care, using Israeli Jewish and Palestinian health professionals, PHR-Israel has operated mobile clinics in the OPT over many years. Most recently, Palestinian health professionals living in Israel have begun working approximately once a month in Gaza as part of a new PHR-Israel initiative.

PHR-Israel has also arranged many meetings with Palestinian government officials in the OPT, petitioned the Israeli government/High Court of Justice for redress, and convened conferences highlighting health care challenges affecting Palestinian health. For example, in November 2019 PHR-Israel and the Palestinian Ministry of Health jointly hosted a conference on mental health in Gaza:

> The conference was introduced by Palestinian officials, Dr. Madhat Mheisen, Undersecretary of Health, Dr. Yihya Khader, Director of the Ministry Department of Health–Mental Health

and Dr. Muhammad Abu Shawish of the Professional Committee on Mental Health. The three speakers expressed deep gratitude to PHRI for its contribution to the mental health field in the Gaza Strip over the past few years and praised the close cooperation between the two bodies.[17]

Evaluating these and many other activities, PHR-Israel has issued many reports highlighting the impact of the Israeli occupation on the health of Palestinians in the OPT. For example, PHR-Israel in 2019 authored a report, "Women's Right to Health in the Gaza Strip," documenting the impact of the closure of Gaza on the health of patients living there.[18] In addition to criticizing the Israeli government, PHR-Israel has been willing to decry the torture of Palestinian prisoners by the Palestinian Authority and Hamas. In its statement "No Struggle Justifies the Use of Torture: The PA & Hamas," PHR-Israel asserted that the PA and Hamas, organizations that "habitually protest against the violence of the Israeli security forces, should also look at the mirror." With these stances, particularly the former, PHR-Israel has come under fire from many segments of Israeli public opinion. Yet it has remained steadfast in its commitment to its mission to "stand at the forefront of the struggle for human rights—the right to health in particular—in Israel and the Occupied Palestinian Territory."[19]

Bridges, The Lancet, and other aspects of health professional PtH engagement via scientific journals

The World Health Organization (WHO) in late 2004 published for several years the magazine *Bridges*. According to the WHO website:

> Israeli and Palestinian health professionals—supported by the World Health Organization (WHO)—have joined together to co-author Bridges—the Israeli-Palestinian Public Health Magazine—in order to help improve the health situation for people in West Bank and Gaza Strip. Bridges, a bimonthly, is a unique publication written, edited, produced and managed jointly by Palestinian and Israeli academics and health professionals under the sponsorship of the WHO. The magazine exemplifies

the WHO paradigm of "Health as a bridge for peace"—the integration of peace-building concerns, strategies and practices with health care—and represents an innovative approach to the planning and implementation of joint projects, sponsored by a professional and impartial body. WHO has launched this innovative tool to bring together Palestinian and Israeli health professionals to address pressing health concerns faced by the people in the region. Bridges: The Israeli-Palestinian Public Health Magazine embodies the exchange of public health information of interest to both Israeli and Palestinian societies, and establishes links between the two communities.[20]

In many ways the magazine reflected the political realities on the ground. While the height of the second intifada had passed by 2005, little evidence of Israeli-Palestinian cooperation around health could be seen either in actuality or as reflected in articles published in *Bridges*. For example, volume 2, number 3 of *Bridges* focused on chronic diseases and contained articles with the following titles: "Chronic Diseases in Palestine: The Rising Tide," by Hani Abdeen, dean of the Al Quds School of Medicine in East Jerusalem (claimed as a future capital by the Palestinian Authority but annexed by Israel in 1980); and "Chronic Diseases in Israel: Current Status and Importance," by Lital Keinan-Boker (deputy director of the Israel Center for Disease Control in the Ministry of Health). No reports of joint ventures between Israelis and Palestinians appeared in this or, in fact, most issues of *Bridges*. Instead, this same issue published an article that consisted of an interview with Alvaro de Soto, the special coordinator for the Middle East Peace Process and the UN Secretary General Personal Representative to the Palestine Liberation Organization and the Palestinian Authority. De Soto opined, "But, if you end up with a political polarization, in which the two parties at the governmental level are essentially not on speaking terms, it makes contacts between civil societies all the more necessary than when governments are on speaking terms.... I would encourage ongoing projects such as Bridges to continue." Yet within a few short years, Bridges ceased operations.[21]

As one of the top three medical journals in the world, The *Lancet*, based in England, has an outsize impact on scientific and, indeed, general opinion. Importantly, it has devoted a great deal of attention to the Israeli-Palestinian conflict since 2000. Richard Horton, its longtime editor, initially took a very different approach to the health implications of the Israeli-Palestinian conflict. In the years after the second intifada, The *Lancet*, with a specific emphasis on health professionals, both sponsored scientific articles and published opinion pieces taking a distinctly pro-Palestinian perspective, as demonstrated in the following statement: "a very powerful determinant of Palestinian health is the State of Israel, whose economic, political, and military superiority continue to be applied, not only to the blockade and recent bombardment and invasion of Gaza, but also to the territorial project within the West Bank."[22] In a dramatic expression of its pro-Palestinian stance, The *Lancet* published an even stronger political opinion piece during one of the Israeli invasions of Gaza (2014):

> On the basis of our ethics and practice, we are denouncing what we witness in the aggression of Gaza by Israel. We ask our colleagues, old and young professionals, to denounce this Israeli aggression. We challenge the perversity of a propaganda that justifies the creation of an emergency to masquerade a massacre, a so-called "defensive aggression." In reality it is a ruthless assault of unlimited duration, extent, and intensity. We wish to report the facts as we see them and their implications on the lives of the people. We are appalled by the military onslaught on civilians in Gaza under the guise of punishing terrorists.... We register with dismay that only 5% of our Israeli academic colleagues signed an appeal to their government to stop the military operation against Gaza.... We are tempted to conclude that with the exception of this 5%, the rest of the Israeli academics are complicit in the massacre and destruction of Gaza.... In addition, in an act that should be understood as a form of solidarity, The Lancet has sponsored to this day regular conferences focused on Palestinian health. The conference proceedings in the form of abstracts continues to be published as a regular feature of The Lancet.[23]

The *Lancet* has continued to publish scientific articles pertaining to the delivery of health services in the OPT and health policy pieces that directly touch on the conflict. One such article from December 2018, "Health and Dignity of Palestine Refugees at Stake: A Need for International Response to Sustain Crucial Life Services at UNRWA," concerned the United Nations Relief and Works Agency for Palestine Refugees in the Near East (UNRWA), which remains responsible for providing care for a significant percentage of the Palestinian population in the OPT.[24] The international response to the challenges confronting the delivery of health services in the refugee camps serving refugee Palestinians (the exclusive role of UNRWA) has varied. The United States, for one, has cut off all funding to UNRWA.

The *Lancet*'s stance explicitly supporting Palestinian rights has not changed, as evidenced by numerous editorials. Most recently, one entitled "Protect Lives before Political Interest in the Middle East," June 2019, declared:

> After cutting support to the UN Relief and Works Agency for Palestine Refugees in the Near East (UNRWA) in 2018 and triggering an unprecedented financial crisis for the agency, Trump is now offering himself as peacemaker in the region, proposing a peace deal based on financial incentives but with no clear pathway to statehood for Palestinians.... What seems to be world leaders' growing shamelessness in using civilian lives as pawns in their proxy war chessboard is most concerning, for the health of civilians in conflict is protected by the Geneva Conventions. World leaders need to stop hiding behind a weak UN Security Council and ensure that protecting civilian lives remains their first priority in conflict.[25]

The *Lancet* has published follow-ups from Palestinians that drive home this perspective:

> Palestinians do not need Israel's help to improve health, yet this seems to be their way of absolving themselves of the responsibility of standing up for truth and justice. The logic is incomprehensible: the Israeli army destroys the health system in the occupied Palestinian territory, and it bombs, shells, and shoots Palestinian civilians. Yet instead of calling for the end of onslaughts on civilians and the end of Israeli occupation and colonization of

Palestinian land, Israeli medical professionals call for collaboration to advance Palestinian health. Not only does this not make sense at all—it is insulting. Palestinians do not want Israeli charity. What Palestinians want is freedom to reconstruct and develop our own society. Palestinians also want and deserve justice and freedom. Only then can peace be achieved.[26]

Accusations of a pro-Palestinian bias has dogged The *Lancet* for years. Most recently, in May 2019, The *Lancet* published a letter from physicians living in Israel requesting that the periodical not take de facto political stances on the conflict: "The future status of the West Bank and Gaza will be determined by ongoing dialogue and negotiation. Within the medical community, it is essential that academic institutions and researchers remain apolitical and do not use publications as a means of identifying with a political agenda."[27] The editor of The *Lancet* has taken the position, in the spirit of the German physician Rudolf Virchow, the founder of social medicine in the mid-nineteenth century, that "The defeat of inequality is an important goal of public health."[28] Largely in response to attacks from Israeli physicians, The *Lancet* has sponsored a parallel series on health care in Israel. In an effort to make connections between the parallel but separate *Lancet* initiatives in Israel and the OPT, Horton concluded:

The health predicament for Palestinians is inexcusable. *The Lancet* has a long-standing commitment to the health of the Palestinian people. Next year, we hold our tenth annual meeting of *The Lancet* Palestinian Health Alliance. We are also committed to working with Israeli colleagues to advance the health of Israeli citizens (eg, our Health in Israel Series, published in 2017). These two initiatives currently run parallel to one another. Is it naive to hope that one day these two streams of work might connect? The health professionals and researchers I know in the PT and Israel are inspiring individuals who have devoted their lives and careers to protecting and strengthening the health of their communities. They want peace. They want justice. It is time to consider how we work more closely together in the common cause of healthy lives for all.[29]

Physical attacks on health professionals

Physical attacks on health professionals clearly contravene the Geneva Conventions.[30] Yet, to put it simply, health professionals and institutions taking care of patients, notably hospitals, have been attacked by opposing sides since time immemorial.[31] However, this tragedy has rapidly accelerated in scope and extent since 2000. As stated in a December 2019 *New York Times* article sadly entitled "Where Doctors Are Criminals":

> The Syrian government considers some health workers enemies of the state.... There was the medical student who volunteered in eastern Aleppo even after his classmates were tortured and killed as a warning.... Each took enormous risks to provide medical care to areas in Syria aligned against President Bashar al-Assad. Some were imprisoned and tortured, evidence of how the nearly 9-year-old conflict in Syria has normalized the criminalization of medical care. Physicians for Human Rights, which has documented the collapse of Syria's health care system, said in a recently *released study* that Mr. al-Assad has successfully made medical assistance given to his enemies a terrorist act.[32]

Chapter 16 in this book highlights attacks against Palestinian health professionals by the Israeli military since the early 2000s. While it is challenging to sort through claims made by the Israeli military that Palestinian health professional have used their neutral status as a cover-up for military activities or the understandable concern that a suicide bomber might be "dressed" as a health professional, there remain enough documented Israeli attacks against Palestinian health professionals to warrant concern and a separate chapter in this book, as this issue impacts the opportunities for PtH.

Recent publications pertaining to PtH

What about health professionals as politicians? Does that fit within the framework of PtH? Does a health professional who takes on a political role have greater political credibility because he is a health professional? There is no question that a significant number of heads of state have been health professionals. Radovan Karadic, former head of the Bosnian Serbs, was a psychiatrist; Ayad Allawi, former Prime Minister of Iraq, was a neurologist; and Bashar al-Assad, the President of Syria, is an ophthalmologist. Within the Israeli-Palestinian sphere, Ephraim Sneh, former Minister of Defense in Israel, was a physician; Mustafa Barghouthi, founder and director of the Palestinian Medical Relief Society, is a physician and ran second to President Abbas in the last elections in Palestine that were held in 2005; George Habash, founder of the Popular Front for the Liberation of Palestine, was also a physician. In a recent article in *Medicine, Conflict and Survival*, "Reinventing the Political Role of Health Professionals in Conflict Prevention and Reconciliation," Salih and his coauthors point out with respect to Sudan that two out of the three periods of democracy in Sudan were led by physicians. The first lasted from 1964 until 1969 and was governed by Al-Tigani Al-Mahi, the father of African psychiatry and a professor of psychiatry. The second, from 1985 to 1989, was initially headed by Al-Gazoli Dafalla, a gastroenterologist. Between these two periods the second coup took place and the first peace agreement was signed, partly as a result of the efforts of the Socialist Women's Union led by Fatima Al-Mahmoud, professor of pediatrics and present chair holder of the UNESCO Chair of Peace for Women and Technology.[33]

This article includes reference to another interesting political event influenced by health professionals. In response to a nonviolent demonstration suppressed violently with live ammunition by the Sudanese authorities, the physicians' union in 1985 led a strike that, after it gathered the support of other unions, was able to bring down the government. Salih and his coauthors brought out other examples and concluded by asking: "Whether this represents a systemic model which can appropriately be adopted by others, or just a collection of 'role models' provided by outstanding individuals, is a legitimate question."[34] While this type of action highlighted by Salih may constitute a "role model," I am of two minds whether it represents a form of PtH. It is likely that part of the impact of the physicians' union came from the social credibility of health professionals. Yet, from what can be ascertained in Salih's article, the physicians' union behaved purely as a political actor and did not explicitly focus on their health professional role. It is my impression that the vast majority of health professionals who become politicians have made minimal use of their professional credibility to advance their political career or enhance their political standing.

While the work of Salih et al. might be considered an expansion of the PtH concept, Izzeldin Abulaish, a Palestinian physician from Gaza currently living in Canada, and Neil Arya, a Canadian family physician, certainly expanded the possible reach of PtH in an article published in *Medicine, Conflict and Survival* in 2017:

> Hatred is a pressing public health issue demanding to be taken seriously by the medical community, the public, governments and other institutions. Hatred is an intense, destructive attitude. Its manifestations are war, disease, violence, and cruelty, symptoms that compromise the health, welfare, and functioning of human beings, both at the individual and population level. The global community must recognize hatred as a public health issue in order to move from the management of hatred, to the active prevention of its root causes.[35]

In their article, Abulaish and Arya press this medicalization of hatred with sections entitled "Hatred and violence as public health issues" and "Hatred as an infectious disease." Recent literature has shown that being the subject of discrimination has health effects similar to adverse childhood experiences such as emotional trauma.[36] Abulaish and Arya conclude their article by arguing, "the global community must recognize hatred as a public health issue in order to move from the management of hatred, to the active prevention of its root causes through promotion, education, and awareness. We must measure it and if unable to prevent it, mitigate it."[37] Abulaish, as part of this engagement, has pointed to his own painful experiences of losing members of his family to an Israeli missile attack during the Israeli Gaza invasion in 2014.[38] The authors do not highlight a specific path forward for such a program, and thus far, few have taken up the cause of hatred as a public health issue.

At an individual level, Palestinian and Israeli health professionals continue to interact with each other.[39] Such interaction has not been encouraged by either Israeli or Palestinian official government entities. Yet such training is ongoing even in the COVID-19 era.[40] This certainly describes a form of PtH, even though it is informal in nature and its exact impact is impossible to ascertain. Moreover, it relies on an asymmetrical relationship between Israeli "experts" and Palestinian "trainees." Recognition of this asymmetry has led to far fewer Palestinians interested in training in Israel, although international funds still exist for this type of interaction.

In another recent article, "Healing under Fire—Medical Peace Work in the Field," in *Medicine, Conflict and Survival*—the foremost journal in this field—Louisa Chan Boegli and Maria Gabriella Arcadu highlight the challenges and, yes, opportunities for PtH in very concrete terms in four conflicts throughout the world in various stages of intensity:

> In all four areas, the word "peace" possessed a highly charged political connotation. Whether or not to engage in peace work very much depended on the context. In Thailand, with an official peace process in place and low intensity level of violence, health professionals were willing to consider, and in some cases even enthusiastic to engage in, health and peace work. In Myanmar, despite an ongoing official peace process, the violent Buddhist–Muslim public discourse and the tensions in Rakhine state made the issue "too hot to handle" by health professionals. In Iraqi Kurdistan, where polarization, political divisions and inequality were on the rise, the concept of health and peace was seen as having the potential to contribute to a more tolerant society and to the development of the region. In Syria, where official peace processes had repeatedly collapsed, the word "peace" had dangerous implications, and was viewed with skepticism.[41]

Extrapolating from the information provided by these authors, it would appear that the Israeli-Palestinian conflict might not be ripe for PtH. There is no official peace process in place, unlike in Thailand. As in Myanmar, the Israel Medical Association and all Israeli health professional groups, with the exception of Physicians for Human Rights-Israel, have certainly felt that the Israeli-Palestinian conflict is either "too hot to handle" or, in fact, take the position of the Israeli government. As already noted above, the Syrian government considers health professionals trying to help both sides to be enemy combatants.

This article, written by health professionals who are not from Thailand, Myanmar, or Syria, indirectly raises an important question: What should be the role of international health professional organizations that are neither Israeli nor Palestinian in the Israeli-Palestinian conflict? Very legitimately, the perspective of a Palestinian quoted above could equally apply to international, not just Israeli, organizations: "What Palestinians want is freedom to reconstruct and develop our own society. Palestinians also want and deserve justice and freedom. Only then can peace be achieved."[42] The next section details how Healing across the Divides has addressed these important questions since its inception.

HATD's perspective and actions since its founding in 2004

What is HATD's theory of change and how does it link with past research on PtH and the engagement of other organizations in PtH, particularly as it pertains to the Israeli-Palestinian conflict? We recognize that there is no end in sight to the long-lasting Israeli-Palestinian conflict. With that in mind, HATD is very much focused on its mission of measurably improving health through supporting community-based interventions proposed and implemented by already existing local groups.

At the same time, our theory of change is to work with local community leadership to improve the capacity of their groups to serve their populations. This, we believe, will increase the leadership and group's ability to function more effectively and assertively in their challenging local political context. It is, obviously, up to already existing groups to decide whether or not to participate in our call for proposals. And once a community group is awarded a grant, its leaders or members can choose to incorporate what they wish into their own managerial processes. The only requirement is that grantees demonstrate measurable improvement in health (or, if no improvement occurred, explain why not), a desired outcome that should be of interest to both the funder and the grantee. After all, they are the ones that have expressed interest in the grant—and, presumably and more importantly, their organizational mission promotes health improvement or improved well-being of the people they serve. In addition, the call for proposal process is extremely elastic in terms of topics that we will consider. Finally, and perhaps most importantly, HATD does not insist that the groups get together and participate in dialogue with each other. Any such insistence on dialogue has met with strong resistance, a position that we respect and agree with.

Our theory of bottom-up change calls for utilizing funds and technical/managerial advice to strengthen already existing community groups led by dynamic but underfunded leaders. Our hope, perhaps naive, is that individuals coming from community groups such as those funded by HATD will be at the forefront of any Israeli-Palestinian peace process—even if it is decades or more away. Through a positive influence on community groups, leading to a measurable improvement in the health of more than 200,000 Israelis and Palestinians to date, we also hope to exert a long-term impact on the communities themselves. Lastly, we believe the individuals served through the community-based grantees will carry through, for themselves, their families, and surrounding communities, long-term changes directly or indirectly influenced by the HATD-supported programs. Thus, we are attempting to embed the humanitarian impulse of health improvement within a long-term community-centered strategy. This is, in part, our short- and long-term PtH strategy.

Additionally, we bring together the community groups that we support, with the proviso that they wish to meet. The Palestinian groups in the OPT have been linking up and the Israeli groups have been convening twice a year for years. These gatherings have led to numerous community groups working together—but only in Israel or only in the OPT, separate from each other. Beginning in 2016, our Israeli and Palestinian representatives have also begun convening joint Israeli (Jewish and Palestinian) and Palestinian groups from the OPT for conversation about shared interests. No Israeli and Palestinian (from the OPT) groups have begun to work together. That is not the intent of the gatherings. Our objective in the cross-border gatherings is simply to foster the intimate and detailed exchange of ideas and programs in a small group setting. It needs to be emphasized that there are virtually no opportunities at the time of this writing for engagement between Israeli and Palestinian groups in the OPT.

These joint meetings pose different challenges for the Israeli and Palestinian community groups. Israeli community groups potentially interested in engagement with the "other" need to confront an Israeli public that is, by and large, content with the current state of the continually expanding Israeli presence or occupation of Palestinian land in the OPT. In addition, they have to contend with significant public relations blowback if they agree to regular meetings with Palestinian groups from the OPT. Palestinian groups in the OPT experience accusations of "normalizing the occupation" from other Palestinians in the OPT if they come face to face with their Israeli counterparts. When meetings take place, it is with the understanding that the results of the meetings are not publicized—for example, no photographs of the encounters are placed on social media. They occur in East Jerusalem, a part of Jerusalem annexed to Israel (without recognition by any other country except the United States). The Palestinian community groups based in the OPT need permission from the Israeli military to come to East Jerusalem. Israeli community groups are not permitted, by Israeli law, to go to those parts of the OPT controlled by the Palestinian Authority. Sadly, in 2019 the Israeli military did not allow any of the joint gatherings to occur.

PtH is a political process. Humanitarian actions, as the Doctors without Borders document quoted above asserted, are explicitly political today. Active or passive HATD decisions have political implications. For example, not all community-based groups are eligible for grants. On the Israeli side, we do not fund any settler groups in the OPT. Given the adamant refusal of the vast majority of settlers to accept an independent Palestinian state, we do not see the Israeli settler movement to be a force for peace. Thus, the HATD Board has decided that, from a PtH perspective, for HATD it is not appropriate to be funding settler groups or Jewish community groups based in the OPT. On the Palestinian side, we do not fund any Palestinian groups in the OPT that do not sign the US State Department antiterrorism pledge or any groups on a State Department list of "terrorist" groups. An accusation of supporting "terrorist" groups would be inappropriate and would immediately lead to our ostracism in the United States.

The HATD board takes no positions on the continual crises that frequently emerge from the Israeli-Palestinian conflict. We've debated this decision many times but, as a small organization, we cannot realistically have any impact on the conflict. Standing in solidarity with one side or the other will not make a difference and would simply expose HATD to unnecessary harassment, from either the Israeli government or the Palestinian Authority.

Finally, there are other populations residing in Israel and the OPT who are neither Israeli nor Palestinian and who tend to be marginalized. The African refugee asylum seekers (RAS) make up one such group that HATD has focused on. These individuals, numbering about 70,000 at the maximum and now numbering almost 30,000, have no rights in Israel and live an extremely marginalized existence. Even though the vast majority come from countries whose populations experienced genocide or major trauma, such as Darfur, virtually no one has been given political asylum. HATD is committed to providing at least one grant at all times to an Israeli group serving the African RAS. This commitment constitutes an example of purely humanitarian engagement without regard to PtH.

Concluding comments pertaining to the current situation that HATD confronts

HATD has kept very much in mind the following perspective of Fiona Fox, a British relief specialist.

> There is a new humanitarianism for a new millennium. It is principled, ethical and human rights-based. It will not stand neutral in the face of genocide or human rights abuses. It will assess the long term impact of each humanitarian intervention on development and peace. It will withhold aid if to deliver it could prolong conflict and undermine human rights. It rejects the traditional principle of neutrality as on the one hand morally repugnant and on the other hand unachievable in the complex political emergencies of the post-Cold War period.[43]

HATD's international humanitarian engagement addresses in part the perspective of the Palestinian health professional who argued earlier in this chapter in favor of "just giving us our freedom." In this chapter, I've tried to argue that measurable improvement in health can be seen as one aspect of freedom. Without health, without the confidence to manage one's own chronic illness, "freedom," however one defines the term, is not possible. HATD is simply not strong enough politically to do more and insist on the end of the occupation of Palestinian territory. That assertion is easy to say and by itself is meaningless. Years ago, shortly after HATD began its work, I received such a request from a Palestinian who belonged to a group of diabetics that the community group we were funding was working with, in Singil in the OPT. At the time, the Israeli army had placed boulders at the entrance to the town that blocked it off from the outside world. I asked the diabetic what more we could do to help, and he forcefully stated: Just tell President Bush to end the occupation. I responded by asking, how can we work together so that your health will improve to the point that you will live to see the end of the occupation? That work, we believe, must involve carefully considered engagement with both Israelis and Palestinians.

As stated by David Rieff:

> Can one do more? Always can one do all the things one would like to do? No, not with the best will in the world. The tragedy of humanitarianism may be that for all its failings and all the limitations of its viewpoint, it represents what is decent in an indecent world. Its core assumptions—solidarity, a fundamental sympathy for victims, and an antipathy for oppressors and exploiters—are what we are … when we are at our best. But there are limits. If one has a terrible disease, one may wish for a cure. But if there is no cure, then no doctor should say "I know what to do for you."[44]

HATD never says to any grantee, to any participant, Palestinian or Israeli, we know what to do for you. HATD's approach to PtH can be looked at from both short-term and long-term perspectives. At a minimum, we want to see measurable improvement in health. By itself and not tied to any other objectives, this HATD activity would be purely humanitarian, with all the challenges summarized in this chapter. Yet, as detailed in this chapter, we have also tried to build on the many perspectives of current and past PtH activists and academics and since 2004 have implemented a long-term philosophy of improving health by strengthening already existing community groups, together with their leadership, in both Israel and the OPT. Part of strengthening community groups is bringing the groups together, as described above. Our dream, as naive as it may be, is that some of these leaders will be tomorrow's political leaders. But in the meantime, we will have measurably improved the lives of over 200,000 marginalized Israelis and Palestinians through the efforts of locally driven community initiatives. Our challenge today is how our activities in Israel and the OPT should evolve in a rapidly changing Middle East. I detail some options in the final chapter.

Notes

1 Healthcare in danger. Declaration by the health care in danger community of concern about the current situation of violence against healthcare. (2020) Available at: https://healthcareindanger.org/resource-centre/declaration-by-the-health-care-in-danger-community-of-concern-about-the-current-situation-of-violence-against-health-care/. Accessed: June 21, 2020.

2 Norwegian Refugee Council. *Challenges to Principled Humanitarian Action: Perspectives from four countries.* Available at : https://www.nrc.no/resources/reports/challenges-to-principled-humanitarian-ac-tion-perspectives-from-four-countries/. Accessed: June 21, 2020.

3 Rieff, D. (2002) *A bed for the night: Humanitarianism in crisis.* New York: Simon and Schuster.

4 Doctors without Borders/Medecins sans Frontieres. *Welcome to MSF-Analysis.* Available at: https://msf-analysis.org/introducing-msf-analysis/ Accessed: June 24, 2020.

5 Doctors without Borders/Medecins sans Frontieres Available at: https://msf-analysis.org/introducing-msf-analysis/. Accessed: June 21, 2020.

6 Rieff, D. (2002) *A bed for the night: Humanitarianism in crisis.* New York: Simon and Schuster, p. 303.

7 Williams, R. as quoted In. Rieff, D. (2002) *A bed for the night: Humanitarianism in crisis.* New York: Simon and Schuster, p. 303.

8 Rieff, D. (2002) *A bed for the night: Humanitarianism in crisis.* New York: Simon and Schuster, p. 307.

9 Dews, F. (2013) What is the responsibility to protect. *Brookings Institution.* Available at: https://www.brookings.edu/blog/brookings-now/2013/07/24/what-is-the-responsibility-to-protect/; Accessed: June 21, 2020.

10 Patrick, S. (2019) The World has lost the will to deal with the worst refugee crisis since World War II. *The Council on Foreign Relations.* Available at: https://www.cfr.org/blog/world-has-lost-will-deal-worst-refugee-crisis-world-war-ii. Accessed: June 21, 2020.

11 U.S. Department of State U.S. Embassy, Jerusalem, Public Diplomacy Section, Notice of Funding Opportunity. P 2. https://il.usembassy.gov/wp-content/uploads/sites/33/APS-Embassy-Jerusalem-FY20–1.pdf. Accessed: June 21, 2020.

12 Rieff, D. (2002) *A bed for the night: Humanitarianism in crisis.* New York: Simon and Schuster, p. 293.

13 Barnea, T., Abdeen, Z., Garber, R., et al. (2000). Israeli-Palestinian cooperation in the health field, 1994–1998. Study Report JDC-Brookdale Institute, JDC-Israel, AJJDC & Al Quds University Also available: www.jdc.org.il/jdcisr. Accessed: June 21, 2020.

14 Peres Center. (2019) *Medicine and healthcare*. Available at: https://www.perescenter.org/en/the-organization/projects/medicine/. Accessed: June 21, 2020.

15 Palestinian nongovernmental healthcare organizations are focused on providing direct care to Palestinians. There are relations with Israeli organizations, particularly Physicians for Human Rights – Israel on health and political issues that impact Palestinians. There are also relations with Israeli hospitals for the care and/or transfer of Palestinian patients to Israeli hospitals. The latter may be seen as a form of PtH.

16 Physicians for Human Rights – Israel. Available at: https://www.phr.org.il/en/department/occupied-territories/. Accessed: June 21, 2020.

17 Physicians for Human Rights – Israel. (2019) Third mental health conference in the Gaza Strip. Available at: https://www.phr.org.il/en/third-mental-health-conference-in-the-gaza-strip/. Accessed: June 21, 2020.

18 Physicians for Human Rights – Israel. *Women's right to health in the Gaza Strip* Available at: https://www.phr.org.il/en/international-womens-day-womens-right-to-health-in-the-gaza-strip/?pr=24. Accessed: June 21, 2020.

19 Physicians for Human Rights – Israel. (2019) *No struggle justifies the use of torture.* Available at: https://www.phr.org.il/en/no-struggle-justifies-the-use-of-torture/?pr=24; Accessed: June 21, 2020.

20 World Health Organization. (2004) New public health magazine by Israeli and Palestinian health professionals addresses the health situation in the West Bank and Gaza Strip. Available at : https://www.who.int/mediacentre/news/notes/2004/np26/en/. Accessed: June 21, 2020.

21 *Bridges, Israel- Palestinian Public Health Magazine.* https://reliefweb.int/sites/reliefweb.int/files/resources/44C875EDC5B60C84492571CA0020861B-who-opt-31may.pdf.

22 Becker, A., Al-Ju'beh, K., Watt, G., (2009) Keys to health: justice, sovereignty, and Self-Determination. *The Lancet.* 373 (9668), pp: 985–987.

23 Manduca, P., Chalmers, I., Summerfield, D., et al. (2014) An open letter for the people in Gaza. *The Lancet.* Available at: https://www.thelancet.com/gaza-letter-2014?code=lancet-site. Accessed: June 21, 2020.

24 Kitamjura, A., Jimbo, M., McCahey, J., et al. (2018) Health and dignity of Palestine refugees at stake: A need for international response to sustain crucial life services at UNRWA. *The Lancet.* 392 (10165) pp: 2736–2744. Available at: https://www.thelancet.com/journals/lancet/article/PIIS0140-6736(18)32621-7/fulltext. Accessed: June 21, 2020.

25 June 2019. Editorial. (2019). Protect lives before political interest in the Middle East *The Lancet.* 393 (10187) Available at: https://www.thelancet.com/journals/lancet/article/PIIS0140-6736(19)31234-6/fulltext p. 2176. Accessed: June 21, 2020.

26 Giacamen, R. (2018) The health of Palestinians. *The Lancet.* 392, p. 2268 Available at: https://www.thelancet.com/pdfs/journals/lancet/PIIS0140-6736(18)32934-9.pdf. Accessed: June 21, 2020.

27 Paul, AG., Asher, E., Stanton, SL., et al. (2019) A call for academic medicine to be politically neutral. *The Lancet* 393 (10183) Available at: https://www.thelancet.com/journals/lancet/article/PIIS0140-6736%2819%2930027-3/fulltext. Accessed: June 21, 2020.

28 Horton, R. (2012) Offline: Dangerous oligarchies. *The Lancet* 379, p. 1688. Available at: https://www.thelancet.com/pdfs/journals/lancet/PIIS0140-6736(12)60688-6.pdf?code=lancet-site. Accessed: June 21, 2020.

29 Horton, R. (2018) The health of Palestinians is a global responsibility. *The Lancet*. 392, p.1612. Available at: https://www.thelancet.com/pdfs/journals/lancet/PIIS0140-6736(18)32773-9.pdf. Accessed: June 21, 2020.

30 International Committee for the Red Cross. *Rule 156. Serious violations of international humanitarian law constitute war crimes.* Available at: https://ihl-databases.icrc.org/customary-ihl/eng/docs/v1_rul_rule156 Accessed: June 21, 2020.

31 Physicians for human rights (2020) PHR documents the deliberate targeting of health care systems and personnel, and advocates to hold violators to account. Available at: https://phr.org/issues/health-under-attack/. Accessed: June 21, 2020.

32 Ewing, J., Shoumali, J. (2019) Where doctors are criminals, *The New York Times*. Available at: https://www.nytimes.com/2019/12/20/world/middleeast/syria-medical-criminalization.html. Accessed: June 21, 2020.

33 Salih, AM., Ahmed, JM., Mohamed, JF., et al. (2016) Reinventing the political role of health professionals in conflict prevention & reconciliation: the Sudanese model. *Med Confl Surviv*. 2016;32(2), pp :153–164.

34 Salih, AM., Ahmed, JM., Mohamed, JF., et al. (2016) Reinventing the political role of health professionals in conflict prevention & reconciliation: the Sudanese model. *Med Confl Surviv*. 2016;32(2), pp:153–164.

35 Izzeldin Abuelaish & Neil Arya (2017) Hatred-a public health issue, *Medicine, Conflict and Survival*, 33:2, pp: 125–130.

36 Takahashi, A., Flanigan, M.E., McEwen, B.S., et al. (2018). Aggression, social stress, and the immune system in humans and animal models. *Frontiers in Behavioral Neuroscience*, *12*, (56). Available at : https://www.ncbi.nlm.nih.gov/pmc/articles/PMC5874490/pdf/fnbeh-12-00056.pdf. Accessed: June 21, 2020.

37 Izzeldin Abuelaish & Neil Arya (2017) Hatred-a public health issue, *Medicine, conflict and survival*, 33:2, p. 130.

38 Abuelaish, I (2011). *I shall not hate: A Gaza doctor's journey on the road to peace and human dignity.* New York: Bloomsbury Publishing.

39 Shuttleworth, K. (2016) The Israelis and Palestinians who work together in peace. *The Guardian*. Available at: https://www.theguardian.com/world/2016/jul/11/israel-jews-arabs-palestinians-work-together-peace Accessed: June 21, 2020.

40 Abu Jahal, E. (2020) Hamas quietly allows Gaza doctors to get COVID-19 training in Israel. *Al Monitor: The Pulse of the Middle East.* Available at: https://www.al-monitor.com/pulse/originals/2020/04/gaza-doctors-coronavirus-training-israel-ramallah.html#ixzz6Kop92CKM. Accessed: June 21, 2020.

41 Louisa Chan Boegli & Maria Gabriella Arcadu (2017) Healing under fire – medical peace work in the field, *Medicine, Conflict and Survival*, 33:2, pp: 131–140.

42 Giacamen, R. (2018) The health of Palestinians. 392, p. 2268 *The Lancet*. Available at: https://www.thelancet.com/pdfs/journals/lancet/PIIS0140-6736(18)32934-9.pdf. Accessed: June 21, 2020.

43 Fiona Fox as quoted by Rieff, D. (2002) *A bed for the night: Humanitarianism in crisis.* New York: Simon and Schuster, p. 314.

44 Rieff, D. (2002) *A bed for the night: Humanitarianism in crisis.* New York: Simon and Schuster, p. 334.

Chapter 16

The impact of the Israeli-Palestinian conflict on Palestinian health care professionals working in Occupied Palestinian Territory

Norbert Goldfield and Heidar Abu Ghosh

Introduction

The past few years have seen a dramatic worldwide rise in limits on, attacks on, and even killings of health care workers trying to provide health care to injured individuals engaged in conflict.[1] In addition, and most tragically, health care workers are increasingly targeted for even providing preventive services such as vaccinations or, in the case of the COVID-19 pandemic, just because they are health care professionals.[2] This chapter, focusing on one conflict, the Israeli-Palestinian conflict, will review limits placed and attacks on Palestinian health professionals that have occurred since 2000 from two different perspectives.

Our first lens will be three recent periods: the first, from 2000 to 2005, roughly covering the second intifada; from 2006 to 2018 encompassing two Israeli incursions into Gaza; and from 2018 to the present. With respect to the latter, we highlight, most notably, the attempts by Hamas and Gazans to force a change in Israeli policy toward Gaza by means of Friday demonstrations, kite burnings, and other actions against Israel, all of which were met with killings and injuries, including of health professionals, our particular concern here. For each of these periods, as our second lens, we will concentrate on three types of impacts on health professionals: injuries and killings of health professionals; damage to health facilities, including hospitals; and Israeli limits on health professionals' ability to study and practice their profession. The latter has posed a particular challenge for graduates of Al-Quds School of Medicine in East Jerusalem (part of the contested Palestinian territory that has been annexed by Israel but is claimed by the Palestinian Authority as the capital of a future Palestine in a two-state solution).

The literature we reference includes third-sector reports, both local and international, United Nations perspectives, and Israeli and Palestinian governmental responses to these limits and attacks on Palestinian health care professionals. In this chapter we detail Israeli limits, including attacks on health care professionals, which, following the Geneva Conventions, should not be occurring.

The second intifada, 2000–2005

During the second intifada, many international organizations investigated Israeli military treatment of Palestinian health professionals, including the killings of health professionals by the Israeli army.[3, 4] As, for example, documented in the *Canadian Medical Association Journal (CMAJ)*, a number of organizations, including Amnesty International Canada, examined the deaths of several Palestinian health professionals, most notably the head of the Palestine Red Crescent Society Emergency Medical Services.[5] As quoted in the *CMAJ* article, the IDF response emphasized the exigencies of war and the attempt by IDF soldiers to do their best under difficult circumstances.[6]

The period of 2006–18: the situation in Gaza, 2006–9

Since the Israeli army evacuated Gaza in 2005, there has been ongoing conflict between Israel and Gaza. In addition, there were several Israeli military incursions into Gaza during this period. Israeli military engagement in Gaza has resulted in the deaths of Palestinian health professionals and other types of limits on Palestinian health professionals. From an early 2009 Amnesty International report:

> Air strike on A-Raeiya Medical Centre and its mobile clinics on 5 January 2009. A-Raeiya Medical Centre is located near Shifaa hospital in Gaza City, in a residential area. There are no governmental or military installations in its vicinity. On 5 January 2009 at 1 a.m., both the centre and its mobile clinics in the car park were bombed from the air. According to testimony from the head of the executive committee of the medical centre, Raed Sabah (collected by Israeli human rights organization B'Tselem): "The centre is

well known, and everybody knows it only provides medical services. It admits more than 100 patients per day, and bears flags with medical symbols. No warning was received before the air strike". The damage to the centre is estimated to be 800 thousand US dollars. The centre provides expert care for internal diseases, a paediatric clinic, gynaecology and obstetrics services, urology, neurosurgery and emergency services. The three mobile clinics belonging to the centre were donations from Spain. They were completely destroyed in the bombing.[7]

Medical personnel attempting to evacuate injured civilians to hospitals have been victims of Israeli attacks. Several ambulances have been targeted by direct gunfire and medical personnel have been seriously injured or killed. According to Physicians for Human Rights-Israel, an attack by helicopter fire on medical personnel on December 31, 2008, left three people dead, including a doctor and medic: "[I]n Jabal Kashif in northeast Gaza a crew set out to offer assistance. While approaching the bleeding victim on foot, they were hit by helicopter fire. Dr. Ihab Madhun, medic Muhammad Abu Hasireh, as well as the injured victim, were killed." In another case, an "[a]mbulance belonging to the Al Awda Hospital was hit by helicopter fire [on 4 January]. Arfa Abd al Daim, a senior volunteer medic was killed and two other medical personnel were critically injured."[8]

The *Manchester Guardian*, in its article on the attacks in Gaza, reported the Israeli response: "The Israeli military declined to comment directly on why more than half of Gaza's hospitals were damaged by Israeli bombing but told the Guardian 'an extensive post-invasion investigation' was under way and that it was looking into allegations that hospitals were targeted during the offensive." The article included a formal statement from the IDF: "The IDF does not target medics or other medical staff. As a part of their training, IDF soldiers receive instructions on identifying and avoiding injury to medical staff in the battlefield. However, in light of the difficult reality of warfare in the Gaza Strip carried out in urban and densely populated areas, medics who operate in the area take the risk upon themselves."[9] The Israeli spokesperson was suggesting that, as in many conflicts throughout the world, the only way Palestinian health professionals could avoid harm to themselves was by abdicating their humanitarian duty of providing health and emergency care to the civilian population that was in urgent need of it.

The period of 2006–18: limits on Palestinian health professionals' ability to practice

During this period, Israeli policies and military measures hampered Palestinian health care professionals' ability to practice in at least two ways. The Palestinian economy, particularly in Gaza, followed (and has never recovered from) a downward spiral, impacting the ability of Palestinian health care professionals to deliver appropriate services. The closure of Gaza has led to a paradoxical economic benefit for Israeli pharmaceutical companies.[10] Secondly, the Israeli occupation of the OPT has led to several types of limits on the ability of Palestinian health professionals to practice and upgrade their training. Most notably, Israel for a period of time refused to recognize the right of graduates from Al-Quds University School of Medicine to at least practice in the area of East Jerusalem—the geographic site of their training. According to an article in the *Washington Post*:

> Since graduating from a local medical school nine years ago, Basel Nassar has been barred from serving his community in East Jerusalem, despite a shortage of doctors there. Like dozens of other Palestinian doctors, Nassar has been caught in the political battle between Israel and the Palestinians over East Jerusalem. Israel captured and annexed the traditionally Arab sector in 1967, a step not recognized by most of the world, while the Palestinians seek it as a capital.... Dozens of Palestinian doctors who graduated from Al-Quds University, a school that has a foothold in East Jerusalem, are caught in the political battle between Israel and the Palestinians over the city's eastern sector. Israel has refused to recognize the university's graduates—a move that could amount to acknowledging the Palestinian claims to East Jerusalem as their capital.[11]

Recently, an Israeli court overturned the Israeli Ministry of Health ban against the practice in East Jerusalem of these Al-Quds medical graduates. Despite this and, reportedly, the position of the Israel Medical Association,[12] until very recently, the Israeli government continued to deny Al-Quds medical school graduates the ability to practice in Israel. Finally, after numerous court battles, Al-Quds medical school graduates with Israeli IDs and who pass Israeli medical examinations have been permitted to practice in Israel.[13]

The period of 2006–18: the situation in Occupied Palestinian Territory, 2014–18

During this period, Israel continued to place obstacles before Palestinian health care professionals seeking to provide first aid to injured Palestinians. The largest number of health professional casualties and damage to health care facilities occurred when intense fighting between Israel and Gaza started again in July and August 2014. A report published by Human Rights Watch (HRW) found "credible information that Israeli forces have unlawfully targeted hospitals, clinics, ambulances, and health workers and that Palestinian armed groups used protected areas in and around schools and hospitals to store weapons and stage attacks." HRW further documented an attack on a hospital in Gaza:

> On July 21, 2014, at about 2:40 p.m., Israeli tanks repeatedly fired on the Shuhada' al-Aqsa Hospital in Gaza while patients and staff were inside. The attacks reportedly resulted in three or four civilian deaths and injured about 40 people, including medical staff and patients. The surgical and intensive care units, as well as two ambulances, were damaged, Palestinian Human Rights Organization Al-Haq said.
>
> In June 2016, the Israeli Military Advocate General responded to complaints submitted by multiple Israeli and Palestinian human rights groups, saying that the incident was still under review.
>
> An investigation by the UN human rights office found the facility was not given advance warning of the attack.
>
> Established in 2001, Shuhada' al-Aqsa Hospital was the only major hospital in the Central district of the Gaza Strip, which had a population of about 260,000. In 2011, the most recent year for which data are available, the hospital's emergency department had more than 90,000 patient visits, and its surgical department admitted 4,521 patients.

An Israel Defense Forces spokesperson told the media that initial investigations into the incident found "that a cache of antitank missiles was stored in the immediate vicinity of the Shuhada al-Aqsa Hospital." However, Israel has not published findings of any additional investigation.

The Military Advocate General has not responded to a February 2017 Human Rights Watch letter seeking more information about its investigation into this incident.[14]

An article in the *Guardian* highlighted possible abuses of health care facilities by Palestinian forces, but there was no way to verify these Israeli accusations, as the Israeli army would not allow independent verification:

> It is crucial that respect for the neutrality of medical space is observed by all armed actors. Rumours persist of Gaza's al-Shifa hospital being used as a Hamas "command centre" and Israel has released footage claiming to show that Hamas commandeered ambulances and launched attacks from hospital compounds during the conflict. If true, these are unacceptable breaches of international law that must be brought to account.
>
> But only an independent investigation that has access to Gaza can verify or dispel these accusations, hence the absurdity of Israel not allowing the UN commission in. The violation of the sanctity of hospitals, whether through military use or targeting, is a war crime either way, and must be scrutinised.[15]

At the same time that the fighting in Gaza was giving rise to injuries to Palestinian health professionals, Palestinian health professionals in East Jerusalem confronted a different set of challenges. To summarize what occurred to one health professional: "Fuad Abid, a volunteer paramedic in the Arab Union of Rescue Services in Jerusalem…. was arrested on April 2nd 2013 while attending a protestor who was hurt when demonstrating near the Damascus Gate. Abid, who was kept in detention overnight, was brought before a judge only the day after. The judge overruled the police claim that Abid was disturbing its work and 'civic order.'"[16] "PHR Israel wrote to the Ministry of Health (MoH) and to the Israeli Medical Association (IMA), requesting they act toward supplying adequate defense to medics working in East Jerusalem and independently investigate Abid's violent arrest." The Israeli government representative responded that "such an investigation is not within the scope of his mandate and that he lacks the investigative capacities when testimonies of civilians and police force contradict."[17] Physicians for Human Rights-Israel (PHR-Israel) documented eight cases in which Israeli forces targeted medics and injured them and one case in which medics were prevented from providing medical assistance to injured protesters during demonstrations in East Jerusalem between April and December 2013.[18] In addition, Palestinian health professionals continued to get caught in the cross fire of civil disobedience and Israeli tear gas fire: In May 2014, a Palestinian physician died of tear gas inhalation as part of a nonviolent civil disobedience.[19]

2018–present: the Gaza demonstrations and resulting death/injuries to Palestinian health professionals; ongoing limits on Palestinian health professionals; ongoing interactions between Israeli and Palestinian health care professionals in the OPT, including Gaza

In March 2018, the "Higher National Commission for the March of Return and Breaking the Siege," a Palestinian, largely Hamas-sponsored entity, began to organize weekly demonstrations along the Gaza-Israel border. Aware of the possibility of violence, especially in Israeli-determined "no-go" zones, the Palestinian Ministry of Health in Gaza and other Palestine health organizations established medical first-aid tents and other treatment facilities at demonstration sites. In the first ten weeks of demonstrations, thousands of demonstrators were injured and many were killed. Officials of the World Health Organization asserted:

> "Healthcare workers must be allowed to perform their duties without fear of death or injury," said the Humanitarian Coordinator Mr. Jamie McGoldrick. "The killing of a clearly-identified medical staffer by security forces during a demonstration is particularly reprehensible. It is difficult to see how it squares with Israel's obligation as occupying power to ensure the welfare of the population of Gaza."

These latest incidents come on top of an already-staggering number of attacks on healthcare personnel reported between 30 March and 27 May: 245 health workers and 40 ambulances have been affected by such attacks, according to data provided by the Palestinian Ministry of Health, the Palestinian Red Crescent Society, PMRS and the Union of Health Work Committees. Many of these were hit by live ammunition.[20]

At the same time attacks against Palestinian health professionals have continued to occur in East Jerusalem to the present. In 2018, Israeli soldiers prevented Palestinian paramedics from attending to injured protesters and assaulted ambulance crews who came to take injured protesters.[21] An elderly woman died from a heart attack while inside the Al-Aqsa Mosque in occupied East Jerusalem after Israeli security forces reportedly prevented a Palestine Red Crescent Society ambulance from reaching her.[22]

Conclusions and strategies for protection of health care workers in the OPT

The networks of organized medicine in Israel and the Occupied Palestinian Territory have little connection with each other. As a consequence, organized medicine in Israel has rarely taken a position on behalf of Palestinian health professionals injured by Israeli fire.[23] Non-state organizations such as Physicians for Human Rights-Israel have collected ample documentation and made valiant efforts to influence opinion on the issue. However, with low membership and little ability to sway Israeli public opinion, their impact on limits placed on Palestinian health professionals has been modest.[24] Partly in response, many Palestinian health care organizations have encouraged a boycott of organized Israeli medical organizations.[25] Yet it should be pointed out that engagement between individual health practitioners on both sides continues, a relationship that can be extended to the institutional level.[26]

A new global coalition of organizations created to protect health care workers worldwide, the "Geneva Call," has brought groups together to put forth a new request to protect health care professionals trying to help injured civilians.[27] The Geneva Conventions, as far back as the first one in 1864, protected the sick and wounded in conflicts. These agreements stipulated that health care institutions and professionals cannot be attacked under any circumstances. Consequently, health care workers providing aid to the wounded should not be impeded, let alone attacked, for providing life-sustaining services. Yet a recent review by Safeguarding Health in Conflict "found almost 1,000 documented attacks [against health care professionals] in 23 countries in 2018 alone. At least 167 health workers were killed and 710 were injured as a result of these attacks. We found that hospitals were bombed or shelled in 15 countries."[28]

In examining what has occurred to Palestinian health professionals since 2000, the authors of this chapter note that unlike in the past, when health care professional action was, to a point, respected, today health care professionals represent a pawn in many conflicts worldwide, including the OPT. The vast majority of articles and reports reviewed document ongoing limits placed on Palestinian health professionals. Both the Israeli government and NGOs supportive of the Israeli government position have rebuffed the extensive work of these articles and reports.[29] Leaders of the Israel Medical Association might assert that the Israeli army is simply responding to Palestinian attacks, including those of health professionals.[30] This chapter documents challenges to such an assertion.

We have two hopes. First, although not optimistic that it will be successful, and despite all the challenges, we hope some of the current worldwide movement toward respect for health care professionals takes root in all conflicts. In this regard, we are encouraged by the type of legislation that was recently introduced in the US Congress that aims to protect health care workers in settings of conflict, which we completely support.[31]

Surely the best guarantee of safety for Palestinian health care professionals is a just solution to the Israeli-Palestinian conflict, our second hope, a prospect that seems further away today than at any time since the conflict began. By means of this chapter, and buttressed by many legal and practical efforts, we and others aim to give visibility to the issue and enhance protection of health professionals. Realistically, a political solution to the Israeli-Palestinian conflict is critically important if Palestinian health professionals are to achieve their dream of providing services to their people.[32] The last chapter explores how Healing Across the Divides could consider being more engaged with the issue of enhancing protection for Palestinian health care professionals. In the meantime, Palestinian health professionals, with the help of sympathetic Israeli health professionals, will continue to try to provide aid to injured Palestinians while attempting to practice in the best way possible.

Notes

1 Healthcare in Danger. (2020) Declaration by the health care in danger community of concern about the current situation of violence against healthcare. Available at: https://healthcareindanger.org/resource-centre/declaration-by-the-health-care-in-danger-community-of-concern-about-the-current-situation-of-violence-against-health-care/. Accessed: June 21, 2020.

2 Massod, S. (2019) Pakistan's war on polio falters amid attacks on health workers and mistrust. *New York Times.* Available at: https://www.nytimes.com/2019/04/29/world/asia/pakistan-polio-vaccinations-campaign.html; Accessed: June 22, 2020.

3 Btselem and Physician for Human Rights – Israel (2003) *Harm to medical personnel the delay, abuse and humiliation of medical personnel by Israeli security forces* Available at: https://www.btselem.org/publications/summaries/200312_medical_personnel_harmed. Accessed: June 21, 2020.

4 Physicians for Human Rights – Israel (2002) *A legacy of injustice a critique of Israeli approaches to the right to health of Palestinians in the occupied territories* Available at: https://www.phr.org.il/wp-content/uploads/2016/06/A-Legacy-of-Injustice.pdf. Accessed: June 21, 2020.

5 Sullivan, P. (2002) Israel criticized after Palestinian MDs shot, killed by soldiers in west bank. *CMAJ* 166(13) p: 1705. Available at: https://www.ncbi.nlm.nih.gov/pmc/articles/PMC116171/pdf/20020625s00030p1705.pdf. Accessed: June 22, 2020.

6 Ibid and Physicians for Human Rights – Israel (2002) *A legacy of injustice a critique of Israeli approaches to the right to health of Palestinians in the occupied territories.* Available at: https://www.phr.org.il/wp-content/uploads/2016/06/A-Legacy-of-Injustice.pdf. Accessed: June 21, 2020. Op cit. P. 78.

7 Amnesty International, Health Professional Network. Air strike on A-Raeiya medical centre and its mobile clinics on 5 January 2009. Available at: https://www.amnesty.org/download/Documents/48000/mde150022009en.pdf. Accessed: June 22, 2020.

8 Amnesty International, Health Professional Network. Health services in Gaza – a worsening situation. Available at: https://www.amnesty.org/download/Documents/48000/mde150022009en.pdf. Accessed: June 22, 2020.

9 Chassay, C. (2009) Under attack: how medics died trying to help Gaza's casualties. *The Guardian.* Available at: https://www.theguardian.com/world/2009/mar/23/gaza-war-crimes-medics. Accessed: June 22, 2020.

10 Anderson, T. and Cooper, T. (2014) Besieging health services in Gaza: A profitable business. Available at: http://corporateoccupation.org/2014/02/18/besieging-health-services-in-gaza-a-profitable-business/. Accessed: June 21, 2020.

11 Greenberg, J. (2012) Premier Palestinian medical school graduates struggle to work in Jerusalem. *Washington Post*. Available at: https://www. washingtonpost.com/world/middle_east/premier-palestinian-medical-school-graduates-struggle-to-work-in-jerusalem/2012/07/15/gJQAlzpDoW_ story.html; Accessed: June 21, 2020.

12 https://www.972mag.com/israeli-court-says-palestinian-doctors-can-work-as-foreigners/89450/.

13 Graduates Of Al-Quds University Turn To AG Mandelblit. *The Yeshiva World*. Available at: https://www.theyeshivaworld.com/news/headlines-breaking-stories/433712/graduates-of-al-quds-university-turn-to-ag-mandelblit.html. Accessed: June 24, 2020.

14 Human Rights Watch. (2017) Hospitals, health workers under attack. Available at: https://www.hrw.org/news/2017/05/24/hospitals-health-workers-under-attack. Accessed: June 21, 2020.

15 Kennedy, H. (2015).The 2014 conflict left Gaza's healthcare shattered. When will justice be done? *The Guardian*. Available at: https://www.theguardian.com/commentisfree/2015/jun/29/2014-conflict-gaza-healthcare-hospitals-war-crime-israel-hamas. Accessed: June 22, 2020.

16 Physicians for Human Rights – Israel. (2013) Disregard the safety of Palestinian medics in East Jerusalem. Abid and Hayat are Palestinian residents of East Jerusalem; They are also Paramedics and Colleagues. Available at: https://www.phr.org.il/en/disregard-safety-palestinian-medics-east-jerusalem/. Accessed to: June 22, 2020.

17 In his response of May 23rd 2013, Prof. Ronnie Gamzu, Executive Director of MOH, stated that such an investigation is not within the scope of his mandate and that he lacks the investigative capacities when testimonies of civilians and police force contradict. His response failed to relate to any responsibility whatsoever for the MOH to defend medical teams in East Jerusalem so they can safely and adequately do their job. IMA had not responded. Physicians for Human Rights – Israel. (2013) Disregard the Safety of Palestinian Medics in East Jerusalem. Abid and Hayat are Palestinian residents of East Jerusalem; they are also paramedics and colleagues. Available at: https://www.phr.org.il/en/disregard-safety-palestinian-medics-east-jerusalem/. Accessed to: June 22, 2020.

18 Amnesty International. Trigger Happy: Israel's use of excessive force in the west bank. http://www.amnesty.org/fr/library/asset/MDE15/002/2014/en/349188ef-e14a-418f-ac20-6c9e5c8d9f88/mde150022014en.pdf.

19 An elderly Palestinian physician has died due to the effects of teargas inhalation. He was hurt and hospitalized several days ago. Local sources said that Dr. Samih Abu Oheish, 64, from Abu Dis Town southeast of occupied Jerusalem, was hospitalized in a critical condition after inhaling gas fired by Israeli soldiers invading the town on Sunday. *Palestine Today* May 27, 2014. Bannoura, S. (2014) Jerusalem physician dies due to effects of teargas inhalation *International Middle East Media Center* Available at: https://imemc.org/ article/67939/. Accessed: June 22, 2020.

20 World Health Organization. (2018) UN agencies deeply concerned over killing of health volunteer in Gaza. Available at: http://www.emro.who.int/ pse/palestine-news/un-agencies-deeply-concerned-over-killing-of-health-volunteer-in-gaza.html?format=html. Accessed: June 22, 2020. See also Medical Aid for Palestinians Gaza Health Workers in the Firing Line. Available at: https://www.safeguardinghealth.org/sites/shcc/files/MAP-Protection-for-Palestinian-Healthcare-Briefing-2018.pdf. Accessed: June 22, 2020.

Médecins du Monde. Violence against healthcare in Gaza Available at: https://www.safeguardinghealth.org/sites/shcc/files/Violence_against_Healthcare_Gaza_2018.pdf Accessed: June 22, 2020.

21 West Bank: Israeli soldiers prevent paramedics from providing first aid (VIDEO) The Palestine Chronicle. Available at: http://www.palestinechronicle.com/israeli-soldiers-prevent-paramedics-provide-first-aid-video/. Accessed: June 22, 2020.

22 Hagbard, C. 68-year-old Palestinian woman dies when Israeli forces block ambulance. *International Middle East Media Center.* Available at: https://imemc.org/article/68-year-old-palestinian-woman-dies-when-israeli-forces-block-ambulance/.Accessed: June 22, 2020.

23 Amnesty International. Under constant medical supervision: torture, ill-treatment and the health professions in Israel and the Occupied Territories. London: AI, 1996. Available at: https://www.refworld.org/docid/3ae6a98620.html. Accessed: July 5, 2020.

    See also: Summerfield D. (2003). Medical ethics, the Israeli Medical Association, and the state of the World Medical Association: Author's response to allegation and to BMA. *BMJ: British Medical Journal, 327*(7423), pp: 1107–1108.

    Blachar, Y. (2003). Medical ethics, the Israeli Medical Association, and the state of the World Medical Association: IMA president's response to open letter to the BMA. *BMJ (Clinical Research ed.), 327*(7423), pp: 1107–1108.

24 We would like to highlight the particularly important role that PHR-Israel has played in obtaining needed care for Palestinians living in the OPT.

25 Palestinian medical and health institutions call for imposing measures against the Israel Medical Association. (2007) Boycott Divestment Sanctions. Available at: https://bdsmovement.net/news/palestinian-medical-and-health-institutions-call-imposing-measures-against-israel-medical. Accessed: June 22, 2020.

26 Shuttleworth, K. (2016) The Israelis and Palestinians who work together in peace. *The Guardian.* Available at: https://www.theguardian.com/world/2016/jul/11/israel-jews-arabs-palestinians-work-together-peace. Accessed: June 22, 2020.

27 Geneva call launches an innovative new deed of commitment on protecting health care in armed conflict. Available at: https://www.genevacall.org/geneva-call-launches-an-innovative-new-deed-of-commitment-on-protecting-health-care-in-armed-conflict/. Accessed: June 22, 2020.

28 Safeguarding Health Coalition. (2018) Impunity remains: Attacks on healthcare in 23 countries in conflict. Available at: https://www.safeguardinghealth.org/sites/shcc/files/SHCC2019final.pdf; Accessed: June 23, 2020.

29 Steinberg, G. and Balanson, N. (2013) NGO malpractice: The political abuse of medicine, morality and science. NGO Monitor. Available at: http://www.ngo-monitor.org/data/images/File/NGO_Malpractice.pdf. Accessed: June 22, 2020.

30 Blachar, Y. (2002) Health toll of the Middle East crisis. *The Lancet*; 359:1859. Available at: https://www.thelancet.com/journals/lancet/article/PIIS0140-6736(02)08682-8/fulltext. Accessed: July 5, 2020.

31 Physicians for Human Rights – Israel. Physicians for human rights PHR-led bill to protect health workers introduced. (2013) Available at: http://physiciansforhumanrights.org/press/press-releases/phr-led-bill-to-protect-health-workers-introduced.html. Accessed: June 22, 2020.

32 Angelo Stefanini and Hadas Ziv. (2004) Health occupied Palestinian territory: Linking health to human rights. *Health and human rights*, 8, (1), pp. 160–176.

Chapter 17

Looking forward

Peace building through health options for Healing Across the Divides

Norbert Goldfield

"What is this optimism?" said Cacambo. "Alas!" said Candide, "It is the madness for maintaining that everything is right when it is wrong."[1]

In fact, I am not an optimist. But I believe that not taking action that has a *realistic* potential of building peace and thus saving lives is not an option. The challenge is how to be engaged while being as effective as possible. To be effective in the Israeli-Palestinian conflict, it is important to make a careful assessment of its current political state and its impact on organizations such as Healing Across the Divides (HATD).

In this concluding chapter, I first make personal observations, based on our work at HATD, regarding the current state of Palestinian and Israeli civil society—that is, the nongovernmental organizations that improve society, the very organizations that HATD engages with. I continue these personal observations into my only explicitly political comments on the Israeli-Palestinian conflict in this book, and how I imagine resolution of the conflict, which will likely not occur in my lifetime. I then ask how HATD could fit within the current Israeli and Palestinian civil society landscape and eventually affect the continuously evolving political stalemate. In my concluding comments, I focus on the relevance of HATD and similar organizations and explore how, considering this political assessment, HATD's impact could continue or maybe even expand.

Palestinian and Israeli civil society

Israeli and Palestinian civil society, as in every other place in the world, is under extreme political and economic pressure. Taking into account this long-term polarizing conflict, Israeli and Palestinian community-based organizations are lucky to obtain funding. If they are so fortunate, they typically focus on the practicalities of meeting the objectives of the grant. They mostly try to ignore to the extent possible the impact of the conflict on their work. The reasons for this focus are different for Israeli and Palestinian civil society organizations. Christine Seibold touched on some of these issues in Chapter 14 of this book. On the Palestinian side, there is an implicit, if not explicit, acknowledgment of the occupation's effect on organizational operations, but most don't want to discuss it, at least not with outsiders. On the Israeli side, a civil society organization hoping for financial support from, typically, American funders needs to be very careful about any political engagement with the Israeli-Palestinian conflict that recognizes Palestinian rights. In addition, Israeli civil society organizations engaged in any way with the Israeli-Palestinian conflict (such as Zochrot, referred to in Chapter 2) have come under extreme pressure from right-wing organizations for years. This pressure, together with many other factors, has resulted in the remarkable situation in Israel today in which the Labor Party, which was in control of Israel for much of Israel's existence, has been reduced to fewer than 5 seats (out of 120) in the 2020 Israeli Knesset, or parliament.

As discussed in more detail in Chapter 15, most Palestinian and Israeli organizations are willing to meet with the other side, provided no publicity is given to the meetings. On the Israeli side, there appear to be no groups that refused to meet with Palestinian groups for political reasons; on the Palestinian side, a small number of groups refused to meet with their Israeli counterparts for reasons pertaining to the Boycott, Divestment and Sanctions movement (BDS);[2] that is, they did not want to meet with Israeli Jews at all.

I believe the focus of Healing Across the Divides should be, in the long term, to increase resilience and organizational strength, while in the short term, to measurably improve the health of as many marginalized sectors of Israeli and Palestinian civil society as possible. In the face of dueling nationalisms, measurably improving health through increased resilience and organizational strength of local groups may not seem enough, and it isn't. Yet I also recognize that, as discussed in chapter 14, it is the leadership of these groups that provide an important key to appreciating the impact of these leaders and the groups that they lead. Max Weber, in particular, together with many others, pointed to the human need for leadership, especially charismatic leadership.[3] The fact that many of the leaders that Christine Seibold interviewed in Chapter 14—and many of them are charismatic—did not want to discuss the conflict reflects another truth to keep in mind. I believe that many of these leaders realize that the work that they are directing builds on other aspects of the society they are engaged with. That is, to quote Robert Musil: "It is always wrong to explain the phenomenon of a country simply by the character of its inhabitants.[4] For the inhabitant of a country has at least nine characters: a professional one, a class one, a geographic one, a sex one, a conscious, an unconscious and perhaps even too a private one; he combines them all in himself but they dissolve him.... "[5] The leaders we fund are trying to thread the needle between different "characters of a country" as they improve the health, and thereby the strength, of the people they serve. In this way they are right now contributing to the possibility of resolution of the Israeli-Palestinian conflict, however distant that may appear today.

The only long-term viable political option

Like all Peace Building through Health (PtH) initiatives and/or organizations, HATD begins with a belief in the "responsibility to protect" individual human beings at the state, organizational, and/or individual level. Yes, as David Rieff maintains, this is a utopian perspective. He points out, "André Malraux said that utopianism is all well and good, if it proceeds from a courageous apprehension of the world as it actually exists."[6] In the spirit of Malraux's "dictum," I look at the world of the Israeli-Palestinian conflict as the founder of Healing Across the Divides and believe that:

a   Both Israelis and Palestinians deserve a land that they can call their own. For example, even the Palestinian Rashid Khalidi writes about how, at this point in history, both Israelis and Palestinians have their own distinct and evolved nationalistic tendencies. As he puts it, "Israeli Jews consider themselves a people with a sense of national belonging in Palestine, what they think of as the Land of Israel, no matter how this transmutation came about."[7]

b   The Israeli government (supported by the Israeli public) has actively settled almost the entire West Bank (Area A, the part "controlled" by the Palestinian Authority, represents only 20% of the land). By the time this book is published, it is possible that Israel will have formally "annexed" parts of the West Bank. Gaza is a virtual open-air jail—not a place that human beings should be forced to live in.

c   A two-state solution with Jerusalem as the capital of an Israeli and Palestinian land appears to be no longer possible. The Israeli political class will never countenance the removal of large numbers of settlers from the OPT. The Israeli public continues to elect governments that are not supportive of a Palestinian state alongside Israel.

d   With the above in mind, the only option I see that can possibly occur is one country for two peoples. At this point in history, such an option is clearly not acceptable to a majority of Israelis.

e   For option (d) to occur, only Israelis and Palestinians (including Palestinians living in Israel[8]) will be able to realize and work out the details of one land for two peoples. To put it differently, a nation-state is a collection of communities such as exists in Israel today (20% of the Israeli population is Palestinian, along with smaller percentages of Druze and other groups); the question is whether a supranational unit composed of national communities is a feasible ambition in the Israeli-Palestinian conflict. As I've stated in chapter 15, neither Israelis nor, especially, Palestinians should look to any international actor for support of a true peace process involving all parties to the conflict. If anything, countries like the United States have consistently supported Israeli occupation and, in fact, annexation of at least parts of the OPT.

This is as specific as I am willing to go in outlining a political option other than to quote the philosopher Isaiah Berlin that any peace between Israelis and Palestinians will be facilitated by leaders committed to a solution that is "logically untidy, flexible and even an ambiguous compromise. [Peace between Israelis and Palestinians] calls for its own specific policy, since out of the crooked timber of humanity, as Kant once remarked, no straight thing was ever made."[9] The question in my mind is: How can HATD facilitate either one land for two peoples or any solution that gives dignity and life to both Israelis and Palestinians? The short answer is strengthening communities through improved health and, over time, providing opportunities for leaders of these communities to get to know each other.

In this problematic political landscape, what are HATD's short- and long-term options?

Internally, the main challenge HATD faces is sustainability. We are a not-for-profit organization based in the United States. As such, we confront three external headwinds in our efforts to maintain sustainability: many would-be donors interested in the approach highlighted in this book are increasingly and understandably devoting scarce resources to the challenges confronting the United States. Second, many of these same individuals see what is going on between Israelis and Palestinians and have thrown up their hands in despair. Third, we live in a COVID-19 era, and once this immediate situation passes, there will be ongoing concerns over pandemics. As of this writing, the implications in some ways are unclear, but several tragedies are evident. In many large countries, notably the United States and China, the political class not only failed its people but, especially in the United States, exacerbated class, racial, and economic divisions purely for political gain. This has resulted in even fewer resources available for community-based interventions to improve health outside the United States.

While these are significant challenges, HATD enjoys significant advantages. Our main asset is that expenses are low, and considering the size of our grants, we have an outsize effect. Simply put, community health interventions are inexpensive, especially given that HATD has access to some of the best researchers in the world who are expert in these areas. If, in addition, we choose carefully the community groups we work with, HATD can have—and, in fact, has had—a dramatic impact on the health of a large number of marginalized Israelis and Palestinians.

If organizations such as ours can remain financially sustainable, there are a number of questions that we need to consider going forward. Israel is a First World country; the OPT is a Third World "territory" under military occupation. Should we continue to fund programs at all in Israel? Should we continue to fund community groups supporting African refugee asylum seekers (RAS)? Should we engage only with community groups that (for example) reject the occupation or are willing to meet with the other? What about settler groups? They are a significant part of the problem; should they be part of the solution? Should we include additional criteria in our funding decisions? For example, on both the Israeli and Palestinian sides, should we give preference to organizations that engage with civil society or participate in the political process? If yes, what should our criteria be? Should we give preference to organizations that are affiliated with a particular party in either Israel and/or the OPT? Should we consider working more actively with either the Israeli or Palestinian governments, singly or together? Should we take positions on political issues? Should we be working with the grantees on political issues—both local and American? Considering the political statements I summarized in (a) through (e) above, how, if at all, should we adjust the outcome metrics that we require as part of the evaluation process?

I respond to the above questions with the following projections about our future. In Chapter 5, I highlight why simple human decency demands that we continue to support Israeli Jewish community groups working to literally save the lives of the African RAS. We must continue that work. Conversely, as I discuss in Chapter 15, I don't see HATD having a role working with settler groups. As of now, only very small groups of Palestinians living in the OPT communicate with settlers.[10] Settler groups are already strong both financially, organizationally, and politically; they are decidedly not "marginalized," a critical part of our mandate.

If one land for two peoples has any chance for success, HATD must continue to fund community groups serving the large number of marginalized individuals in Israel. Yet we should consider refining our funding criteria. Ideally, the community groups should be willing to undertake civil society initiatives that engage with the "other," especially, for Israeli grantees, with Palestinians—but not from a perspective of inequality or dependency. A key to tying our work to any political outcomes as described above is to focus our projects on initiatives that increase self-confidence and self-reliance, particularly for Palestinians living in the OPT. If one is self-confident regarding one's own health, one can build up resilience. This resilience can serve as a reservoir of strength against the psychic traumas alluded to and specifically highlighted throughout this book. As Dina Nasser, who works at a hospital in East Jerusalem, stated: "just finding the resilience to live a normal day-to-day life under constant harassment is hard enough."[11] HATD should seek out initiatives, both in Israel and the OPT, to measurably build resilience as part of our efforts to measurably improve overall health using community-based interventions.

It is to be hoped that with a programmatic focus at the individual level on improved resilience and confidence, HATD will redouble its efforts to bring community groups together. This may be one of the few positive spin-offs of the COVID-19 era: bringing community-based organizations together virtually, instead of physically, could be an icebreaker. To get beyond that, however, HATD could consider a more political approach to its funding. That is, for example, we could consider funding only Israeli organizations that reject the occupation. Or, playing devil's advocate, one could argue that we should not insist on this red line. Maybe we should restrict ourselves to funding organizations that are willing to at least meet together (without any fanfare or publicity). We will need to explore all options as we combine our insistence on measurable improvement in health together with a political commitment to change in the Israeli occupation.

What should the attitude of HATD be toward the Israeli government and the Palestinian Authority? The Israeli government and the PA have adopted several HATD-funded initiatives that led to improvements in the health of participants during the period of our grant. However, we did not work directly with them on this. We have no engagement with the political authority in Gaza, something that would contravene American law. At the same time, we appreciate Doctors without Borders/Médecins sans Frontière's perspective that "putting the host government in overall charge of aid in conflict situations creates a strain on impartiality, as the state is one of the belligerents in ongoing violence."[12] I believe that we should continue to "thread the needle" by working indirectly with both governments via community groups, encouraging the adoption of our programs, as we have since 2004, while not de facto becoming part of the occupation of Palestinian territories. While many may think we cannot balance these competing interests, I am hopeful that if we, at the board level, and with our grantees, continually dialogue about how to tie grants to the end goal of one state for two peoples, we can work with both the Israeli and PA governmental entities. Maybe we can even envision a situation in which we are funding an initiative—for example, in child safety or breast cancer—that brings both governments (not private groups that are typically extremely marginalized in their own societies) together. Such an endeavor would have to recognize both sides on equal terms, not as in the typical grant in which Palestinians are benefiting from Israeli largesse or technical expertise.

Concluding comments

A focus on improving economics or material well-being is not sufficient; improving health can be a true bridge for peace. Referring back to the very beginning of this book, "Health as a Bridge for Peace (HBP)", as originally defined by the 51st World Health Assembly,

> supports health workers in delivering health programs in conflict and post-conflict situations and at the same time contributes to peace-building. The Health as a Bridge for Peace concept is rooted in values derived from human rights and humanitarian principles as well as medical ethics. It is supported by the conviction that it is imperative to adopt peace-building strategies to ensure lasting health gains in the context of social instability and complex emergencies. We as health professionals recognize responsibilities to create opportunities for peace.[13]

Healing Across the Divides' approach to peace building through health can be looked at from both short-term and long-term perspectives. At a minimum, we wish to fulfill our mission—to measurably improve health through locally driven community health interventions. We have also implemented, since our founding in 2004, a long-term philosophy of strengthening already existing community groups, including their leadership, in both Israel and the Occupied Palestinian Territory. Part of strengthening community groups is bringing the groups together. With this strategy, we have measurably improved the lives and health of more than 200,000 marginalized

Israelis and Palestinians utilizing these locally driven community health initiatives.

Saving a life—the essence of humanitarianism and the essence of being a health professional—is a linchpin of PtH. Yet even humanitarianism represents a political statement. As Doctors without Borders/Médecins sans Frontières (MSF) recently stated in its 2020–23 planning document: "While it is clear that MSF is not driven by political interests, our medical humanitarianism is deeply political. This is because we impartially provide treatment, alleviate suffering and restore dignity to those whose basic existence is under threat by the prevailing political order."[14]

From a political point of view, HATD is guided, short term, by measurable improvements in health; medium term, by building up community groups and the leaders of these groups; long term, by our dream that some of these community leaders will work together to make compromises among themselves in the realization that one state for two peoples is one of only a very few ways forward. The key word is "compromise." In an April 2019 editorial, Richard Horton, the editor of the *Lancet*, highlights the importance of compromise:

> The late novelist, Amos Oz, in *How to Cure a Fanatic* (2012), argued that a "painful compromise" was the only solution to the competing claims of Israel and Palestine. "For me," Oz wrote, "the word compromise means life … the opposite of compromise is fanaticism and death." Expanding on this, Avishai Margalit (*On Compromise and Rotten Compromises*, 2010) writes, "We should, I believe, be judged by our compromises more than by our ideals and norms. Ideals may tell us something important about what we would like to be. But compromises tell us who we are."[15]

In most cases, peacemaking requires bottom-up processes in which groups and individuals publicly support the ideas of peace building and act to persuade their political leaders. But it also requires top-down processes in which emerging political leaders join efforts or initiate peacemaking processes and work to persuade members of society of the necessity of a peaceful settlement of the conflict. A Palestinian colleague privately observed that either top-down or bottom-up scenarios of peacemaking or peace building in the Israeli-Palestinian conflict can occur only when both Israelis and Palestinians believe that there is

- *equality between partners, including equal rights between Israelis and Palestinians*
- *mutual respect between the two conflicting parties*
- *absence of dependency*
- *a clear agenda to develop the weak partner to a level close to the stronger one*
  Partners should work together to stop the humiliation, oppression, and suffering of their counterparts. Are all partners ready to do that?

Put differently, practically speaking, compromise means that Israelis and Palestinians each legitimize the other. This has not happened yet to either the political class or the active citizenry in either Israel or the OPT. The big step will need to be taken by Israelis, because they have de facto control of the OPT. However, I contend throughout this book that this will not occur until Palestinian civil society becomes as organizationally strong as their Israeli counterparts.

Healing Across the Divides staff will never insist that Israelis and Palestinians work together and thus sacrifice their dreams. We only bring community groups together that are objectively committed to improving the health of the populations they serve. We also bring the leaders of community groups together in the fervent hope that by meeting face to face with the "other," the leaders will consider compromising on their national dream while acknowledging the traumas caused by this conflict. Yet a key part of our political approach is to strengthen/empower Palestinian groups and leadership to the extent that the compromises, if and when they occur, can transpire between two equally strong parties. Is this naive? Maybe. But the alternative of doing nothing is not acceptable. This book, I hope, has demonstrated one path to compromise in the Israeli-Palestinian conflict—one via health, the dream of every human being.

Notes

1 Voltaire (1759). Candide chapter 19 verse 5. New York Public Library. Available at: http://candide.nypl.org/text/chapter-19.
2 See https://bdsmovement.net/ for more information on the Boycott Divestment and Sanctions movement.

3 Weber, Maximilian. (1947) *Theory of Social and Economic Organization.* Chapter: "The Nature of Charismatic Authority and its Routinization" translated by A. R. Anderson and Talcott Parsons.

4 I interpret character in this context to be the "national character" reflecting the dueling nationalisms discussed in this book.

5 Musil, R. (1980) *The Man Without Qualities.* Trans Wilkins, E. and Kaiser, E., p. 34 as quoted in Weinstein, F. (1990). *History and theory after the fall.* Chicago: University of Chicago Press. pp. 2–3.
   See Weinstein F for a much more complete theoretical discussion of the relationship between leadership and national characters.

6 Rieff, D. (2002) *A bed for the night.* New York: Simon and Schuster, p. 24.

7 Khalidi, R. (2020) *The hundred years' war on Palestine.* New York: Metropolitan Books. p. 245.

8 International Crisis Group has published reports opining that Palestinians living in Israel may be the key to peace in the Israeli-Palestinian conflict. https://www.crisisgroup.org/who-we-are/people/nathan-thrall.

9 Berlin, I. (1969) *Four essays on liberty.* New York: Oxford University Press, pp: 39–40.

10 Brynt, CC. (2015) Ali Abu Awwad chose nonviolence over revenge. *Christian Science Monitor.* Available at: https://www.csmonitor.com/World/Making-a-difference/2015/0612/Ali-Abu-Awwad-chose-nonviolence-over-revenge.

11 Devi, S (2019) Health in Israel and the OPT in the lead-up to elections *The Lancet* 393 (10175), pp: 973–974 Available at: https://www-sciencedirect-com.ezproxy.library.tufts.edu/science/article/pii/S0140673619305367.

12 Magone, C., Neuman, M., Weissman, F. (2011) Humanitarian negotiations revealed: The MSF experience United Kingdom: Hurst, p. 2. See epilogue in particular. Available at: https://b-ok.cc/book/2574602/1f9eac. Accessed: July 5, 2020.

13 *Health as a Bridge for Peace was formally accepted by the 51st World Health Assembly in May 1998 as a feature of the 'Health for All in the 21st Century' strategy.* Available at: https://www.who.int/hac/techguidance/hbp/about/en/ Accessed: June 23, 2020.

14 Whittall, J. (2019) *Medical humanitarian needs in a changing political and aid environment* Médecins sans Frontières. Available at: http://msf-analysis.org/medical-humanitarian-needs-changing-political-aid-environment/. Accessed: June 23, 2020.

15 Horton, R. (2019) Offline: The case for compromise *The Lancet* vol. 393 (10181), p. 1582. Available at https://www.thelancet.com/journals/lancet/article/PIIS0140-6736(19)30890-6/fulltext. Accessed: June 22, 2020.

Appendix

List of organizations that Healing Across the Divides has worked with and a brief description of their intervention

One in Nine Increase breast cancer awareness among ultra-Orthodox Jewish women in Israel

Ahli Balatah Al-Balad Club (ABBC) Improve the health of diabetics in the Nablus area in the West Bank, Occupied Palestinian Territory (OPT)

Al-Maqdese for Society Development Drug abuse prevention among Palestinian youth in East Jerusalem

Al-Tufula Promote nutrition-based wellness and expansion of health rights for Arab women in northern Israel

Al-Manal/Kokhav/Mifras B Galil Improve mental and physical health among disabled Jewish and Palestinian young women living in northern Israel

ASSAF (Aid Organization for Refugees and Asylum Seekers in Israel)/Israel AIDS Task Force (AITF) HIV counseling and preventive services among African refugee asylum seekers (RAS) in Israel

Beit Natan Increase breast cancer awareness among ultra-Orthodox Jewish women in Jerusalem, Israel

Bet Shemesh Health rights among Jewish people in Bet Shemesh, Israel

Beterem Decrease childhood accidents at home by working through community-engaged grandmothers in northern Israel

Caritas Chronic Disease Self-Management for individuals with chronic illness in the Ramallah area, OPT

Dar Al-Kalima Health and Wellness Center Expand health and wellness through exercise and nutrition for young women in the Bethlehem district of the OPT

Diabetes Palestine Chronic Disease Self-Management for individuals with Type 1 diabetes in Gaza, OPT

Family Defense Society (FDS) Chronic Disease Self-Management for women with obesity in the Nablus area, OPT

Friends by Nature Use local gardens to help Ethiopian Jewish women in Israel improve their health through nutrition

Galilee Society Chronic Disease Management for Palestinians with Type 2 diabetes in northern Israel

Hadassah Optimal Increase nutrition and exercise among young mothers and their children in Israel

Hiyot Working with Ethiopian Jewish teens and mothers on issues of sexual health and well-being in Israel

Ilabun Promote women's health and wellness for Arab communities in northern Israel

Israel Association of Community Centers Promote women's health and health awareness for Orthodox women outside Jerusalem, Israel

Jerusalem African Community Center Alleviate post-traumatic stress disorder and depression among RAS in Jerusalem, Israel

Kayan Feminist Organization Expand health rights of Palestinian women in northern Israel through civic engagement

Kuchinate Improve resilience and economic support for African RAS, Tel Aviv, Israel

Ma'an Increase awareness of domestic violence among Bedouin women and offer support to victims of domestic violence in the Negev, southern Israel

Mesila Promote sexual health among Ethiopian Jewish youth, near Haifa, Israel

Ne'eman Increase awareness about the risks of stroke among women in Israel

Palestinian Medical Relief Society Chronic Disease Management among Palestinians with Type 2 diabetes in the Ramallah area, OPT

Palestinian Working Women Society for Development Build resilience among Palestinian women and teenage girls in the southern OPT

Physicians for Human Rights-Israel Expand health promotion activities among marginalized Russian women in Beersheva, Israel

Rahat Engage with Bedouin women in southern Israel about the importance of healthy lifestyle habits

Sha'ab Genetic counseling among Palestinians living in northern Israel

Tene Briut Chronic Disease Management among Ethiopian Jews with Type 2 diabetes in northern Israel

White Hill Farm Joint urban farming venture between the towns/villages of Rachmeh and Yeroham in southern Israel

Women Against Violence Promote women's health rights among Arab women in Nazareth and the Galilee in northern Israel

Women's Studies Centre (WSC) Provide psychological support to Palestinian women living in East Jerusalem and Silwan

Yasmin El Negev Empower Bedouin women in Israel to create social change impacting the overall well-being of their community

Yes Theatre Use drama therapy to build resilience among Palestinian women and teenagers in the southern OPT

Contributing authors

1. **Abu Ghosh, Heidar.** Ramallah, OPT. Chapter 16. kteish@yahoo.com;

2. **Anabtawi, Rafa.** Kayan Feminist Organization, Haifa, Israel. Chapter 9. rafa@kayan.org.il;

3. **Calif, Elad.** Beterem, Tel Aviv, Israel. Chapter 6. eladc@beterem.org;

4. **Constantini, Naama.** Heidi Rothberg Sports Medicine Center, Shaare Zedek Medical Center, Hebrew University, Jerusalem, Israel. Chapter 8. naamacons@gmail.com;

5. **Goldfield, Norbert.** American not-for-profit Healing Across the Divides, USA. Chapters 1, 2, 3, 4, 5, 6, 7, 9, 10, 11, 12, 13, 15, 16, 17. norbert@healingdivides.org

6. **Hasan, Nael.** National Rehabilitation Center, Abu Dhabi, United Arab Emirates. Chapter 4. naelm68@gmail.com;

7. **Jwihan, Isam.** Al-Maqdese for Society Development, East Jerusalem, Palestinian Authority. Chapter 4. isamjwe@gmail.com;

8. **Katzen, Zoe.** Kayan Feminist Organization, Haifa, Israel. Chapter 9. zoe@kayan.org.il;

9. **Khatib, Mohammed.** The Galilee Society, Tamra, Israel. Chapter 3. khatib.health@gmail.com;

10. **Malkin, Gali.** Beterem, Tel Aviv, Israel. Chapter 6. galim@beterem.org;

11. **Monsoor, Anwar.** Kayan Feminist Organization, Haifa, Israel. Chapter 9. mona@kayan.org.il;

12. **Muhsin, Gada.** Al-Maqdese for Society Development, East Jerusalem, Palestinian Authority. Chapter 4. gada@al-maqdese.org;

13. **Orr, Daniela.** Beterem, Tel Aviv, Israel. Chapter 6. danielao@beterem.org;

14. **Polak, Rani.** Institute of Lifestyle Medicine, Department of Physical Medicine and Rehabilitation, Harvard Medical School, Spaulding Rehabilitation Hospital, Boston, MA, USA; Lifestyle Medicine Center, Sheba Medical Center, Tel Hashomer, Israel. Chapter 8. Rani.Polak@sheba.health.gov.il;

15. **Rawson, Richard A.** Vermont Center for Behavior and Health, Lerner School of Medicine, University of Vermont, 1 South Prospect St., Burlington, VT, USA, and Integrated Substance Abuse Programs, Geffen School of Medicine, University of California at Los Angeles. Chapter 4. rrawson@mednet.ucla.edu;

16. **Seibold, Christine.** Business Coach, Founder of Fremprendedoras, Miami, Florida. Chapter 14. christineseibold6003@gmail.com;

17. **Shehada, Safa.** Ma'an Consultant. Lod, Israel. Chapter 10. safa.maan@gmail.com;

18. **Stein-Zamir, Chen.** Ministry of Health, Jerusalem District Health Office, Israel. Chapter 8. chen.zamir@lbjr.health.gov.il;

19. **Verbov, Gina.** The Hebrew University of Jerusalem Faculty of Medicine, the Hebrew University, and Hadassah Braun School of Public Health and Community Medicine, Jerusalem, Israel. Chapter 8. gina.leib@lbjr.health.gov.il.

Index

PGIL2023USA